Practical Urodynamics for the Clinician

Andrew C. Peterson • Matthew O. Fraser
Editors

Practical Urodynamics for the Clinician

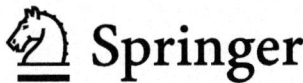 Springer

Editors
Andrew C. Peterson, MD
Department of Surgery
Division of Urology
Duke University Medical Center
Durham, NC, USA

Matthew O. Fraser, PhD
Department of Surgery
Division of Urology
Duke University Medical Center
Durham, NC, USA

ISBN 978-3-319-20833-6   ISBN 978-3-319-20834-3   (eBook)
DOI 10.1007/978-3-319-20834-3

Library of Congress Control Number: 2015952627

Springer Cham Heidelberg New York Dordrecht London
© Springer International Publishing Switzerland 2016
This work is subject to copyright. All rights are reserved by the Publisher, whether the whole or part of the material is concerned, specifically the rights of translation, reprinting, reuse of illustrations, recitation, broadcasting, reproduction on microfilms or in any other physical way, and transmission or information storage and retrieval, electronic adaptation, computer software, or by similar or dissimilar methodology now known or hereafter developed.
The use of general descriptive names, registered names, trademarks, service marks, etc. in this publication does not imply, even in the absence of a specific statement, that such names are exempt from the relevant protective laws and regulations and therefore free for general use.
The publisher, the authors and the editors are safe to assume that the advice and information in this book are believed to be true and accurate at the date of publication. Neither the publisher nor the authors or the editors give a warranty, express or implied, with respect to the material contained herein or for any errors or omissions that may have been made.

Printed on acid-free paper

Springer International Publishing AG Switzerland is part of Springer Science+Business Media (www.springer.com)

Preface

Urodynamics have sometimes been considered to be confusing, ambiguous, and complex. However, with increasing improvements in technology, software, and equipment, this heretofore often perplexing series of tests has become significantly simplified for use by the clinician in today's busy urologic practice.

Many textbooks on this subject have relied heavily on long descriptions of the basic science of urodynamics and complex physiology. However, urodynamics in today's clinical world may produce very practical and clinically relevant data with significant impact on patient care. The objective of this book is to offer the reader a guide to the preparation, conduct, and interpretation of these studies in the everyday clinical scenario.

One must remember that the term urodynamics actually refers to a series of simple tests that are designed to be combined to produce useful information for a particular clinical situation. Very much like a high-performance race car engine is a complex and confusing machine, urodynamics can be thought of as a combination of multiple simple machines put together for a specific purpose. For instance, a radiator, a carburetor, fuel injector, and piston are all subcomponents of the complex car engine that when working in unison form a smooth well-running powerful device. In much the same manner, the urine flow, postvoid residual, cystometrogram, and EMG when combined together will give the clinician powerful data to apply to the specific clinical question at hand. It's also important to remember that one does not need to include all of the subcomponents in order to address a specific concern about a patient's complaint. For instance, one may only need noninvasive urodynamics (uroflow/postvoid residual) in one clinical scenario, while another may require a complex study with the combination of the cystometrogram, EMG, fluoroscopy, and pressure flow studies.

We have arranged this book into these components as outlined above. The book starts with a basic physiology section focusing on the relevant principles and equations needed for practical clinical urodynamics. The reader is then taken on a tour of all of the individual tools of urodynamics starting with noninvasive urodynamics, the cystometrogram, the pressure flow study, the EMG, and the use of fluoroscopy. In addition, we have included chapters with practical relevance to the clinician such as a description of the type of equipment needed to start a urodynamics lab, the use of the currently available nomograms, and a chapter on the special population of children. With the goal of this being primarily a handbook for use by the clinician, there is not a lot of discussion within this textbook about specific diagnoses and treatment.

We hope that clinicians and current learners of urology such as residents and fellows will be able to obtain the required practical knowledge about equipment, the type of testing, and the performance of this testing to become proficient in this important study.

I sincerely appreciate all the hard work the authors have provided for this great textbook—they are all busy clinicians and pioneers in the field of both urodynamics and voiding dysfunction/incontinence. To Dr. George Webster, I owe an enduring debt of gratitude for his medical training, mentorship, and support throughout my time both running our urodynamics laboratory at Duke and in production of this textbook.

Durham, NC, USA

Andrew C. Peterson
Matthew O. Fraser

Contents

The Basic Science Behind Practical/Clinical Urodynamic Analysis 1
Matthew O. Fraser

Urodynamics Equipment: What the Clinician Needs to Know to Set Up the Lab 9
Andrew P. Windsperger and Brian J. Flynn

The Clinical Evaluation of the Patient Who Requires Urodynamics 21
Maria Voznesensky and R. Clay McDonough III

Noninvasive Urodynamics 31
Oscar Alfonso Storme and Kurt Anthony McCammon

The Cystometrogram 43
Ryan L. Steinberg and Karl J. Kreder

The Pressure Flow Study 61
Kirk M. Anderson and David A. Hadley

The EMG 77
Kristy M. Borawski

The Use of Fluoroscopy 89
Tom Feng and Karyn S. Eilber

Putting It All Together: Practical Advice on Clinical Urodynamics 101
Julian Wan and John T. Stoffel

Nomograms 113
David Jiang and Jennifer Tash Anger

Ambulatory Urodynamics 125
Paholo G. Barboglio Romo and E. Ann Gormley

Bedside Urodynamics 135
Andrew C. Peterson

Practical Urodynamics in Children 143
Sherry S. Ross and John S. Wiener

Index 161

Contributors

Kirk M. Anderson, M.D. Department of Urology, University of Colorado, Aurora, CO, USA

Jennifer Tash Anger, M.D., M.P.H. Division of Urology, Department of Surgery, Cedars-Sinai Medical Center, Beverly Hills, CA, USA

Kristy M. Borawski, M.D. Department of Urology, University of North Carolina—Chapel Hill, Chapel Hill, NC, USA

Karyn S. Eilber, M.D. Division of Urology, Department of Surgery, Cedars-Sinai Medical Center, Beverly Hills, CA, USA

Tom Feng, M.D. Department of Surgery, Division of Urology, Cedars-Sinai Medical Center, Los Angeles, CA, USA

Brian J. Flynn, M.D. Department of Surgery/Urology, University of Colorado Denver, Aurora, CO, USA

Matthew O. Fraser, Ph.D. Department of Surgery, Division of Urology, Duke University Medical Center, Durham, NC, USA

E. Ann Gormley, M.D. Section of Urology, Department of Surgery, Dartmouth-Hitchcock Medical Center, Mary Hitchcock Hospital, Lebanon, NH, USA

David A. Hadley, M.D. Loma Linda Urology, Loma Linda University Medical Center, Loma Linda, CA, USA

David Jiang, B.A., M.S. Oregon Health and Science University, Department of Urology, Portland, OR, USA

Karl J. Kreder, M.D. Department of Urology, University of Iowa, Iowa City, IA, USA

Kurt Anthony McCammon, M.D. Department of Urology, Eastern Virginia Medical School, Virginia Beach, VA, USA

R. Clay McDonough III, M.D. Department of Urology, Maine Medical Center, South Portland, ME, USA

Andrew C. Peterson, M.D. Department of Surgery, Division of Urology, Duke University Medical Center, Durham, NC, USA

Paholo G. Barboglio Romo, M.D., M.P.H. Section of Urology, Department of Surgery, Dartmouth-Hitchcock Medical Center, Lebanon, NH, USA

Sherry S. Ross, M.D. Department of Urology, The University of North Carolina at Chapel Hill, Chapel Hill, NC, USA

Ryan L. Steinberg, M.D. Department of Urology, University of Iowa, Iowa City, IA, USA

John T. Stoffel, M.D. Division of Neurourology and Pelvic Reconstructive Surgery, Department of Urology, University of Michigan Medical Center, Ann Arbor, MI, USA

Oscar Alfonso Storme, M.D. Department of Urology, Eastern Virginia Medical School, Virginia Beach, VA, USA

Maria Voznesensky, M.D. Department of Urology, Maine Medical Center, South Portland, ME, USA

Julian Wan, M.D., F.A.A.P. Division of Pediatric Urology, Department of Urology, C.S. Mott Children's and Von Voigtlander Women's Hospital, Ann Arbor, MI, USA

John S. Wiener, M.D. Division of Urologic Surgery, Department of Surgery, Duke University Medical Center, Durham, NC, USA

Andrew P. Windsperger, M.D. Department of Urology, St. Cloud Hospital, CentraCare Health, Adult and Pediatric Urology of Sartell, Sartell, MN, USA

The Basic Science Behind Practical/Clinical Urodynamic Analysis

Matthew O. Fraser

The Lower Urinary Tract

Function

The function of the lower urinary tract is to collect and store urine, and then to periodically expel urine when the bladder is full and the situation is environmentally appropriate. **One of the hallmarks of mammalian evolution is the development of a urinary bladder-urethral complex, rather than the bladder emptying directly into a cloaca.** Although the bladder is the primary organ of urine storage and generates the pressure to evacuate urine, the urethra, a relatively recent evolutionary development, actively participates both in storage and release functions as well. The actions of these structures are coordinated through reflexes involving the spinal cord and brainstem, with inhibitory control exerted from higher cortical centers [1].

Anatomy

The lower urinary tract comprises the distal ureters, the trigone, the urinary bladder and the urethra. The ureters enter the bladder base and merge with the trigone. The trigone is a specialized region of intercalated ureteral and bladder smooth muscle [2] that extends dorsally down the proximal urethra.

M.O. Fraser, Ph.D. (✉)
Department of Surgery, Division of Urology, Duke University Medical Center, 508 Fulton Street, Durham, NC 27705, USA
e-mail: matthew.fraser@duke.edu

© Springer International Publishing Switzerland 2016
A.C. Peterson, M.O. Fraser (eds.), *Practical Urodynamics for the Clinician*, DOI 10.1007/978-3-319-20834-3_1

The bladder itself is a saccular muscular structure with greatest compliance laterally and ventrally [3]. The bladder muscle is referred to as the detrusor and is organized as a single layer of randomly oriented fibers at the dome which organizes into a three layer system at the base [4]. The longitudinal muscle layers (internal and external) surround the central circular smooth muscle layer. The bladder pattern extends into the mid-length of the intrapelvic urethra, with the inner longitudinal layer extending to 2/3 of the length from the bladder base [5]. Because these smooth muscle layers are continuous between the bladder and urethra, the term vesicourethral muscularis has been used to describe the bladder-urethral unit [6].

Perhaps the most defining characteristics of the urethra is the circumferential smooth muscle layer, which is very thin in the bladder but much more prominent in the urethra [5], the external layer of circumferential striated muscle (the rhabdosphincter), and that it passes through the pelvic floor. In females it opens directly to the external environment in the vulvar vestibule. In males it traverses the ventral penis.

Figure 1 presents a highly stylized diagram of the vesicourethral muscularis and rhabdosphincter to illustrate the muscle layers (components not drawn to scale, outer longitudinal layer not included).

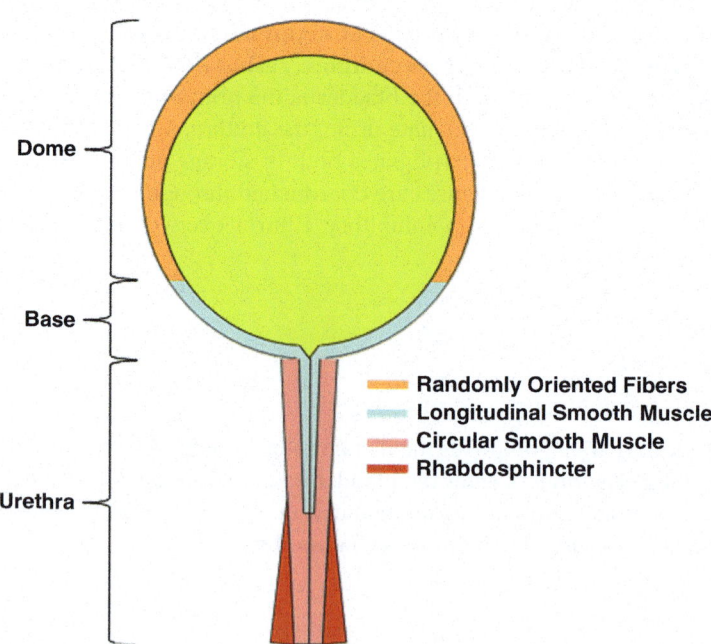

Fig. 1 Highly stylized diagram of the vesicourethral muscularis and rhabdosphincter to illustrate the muscle layers (components not drawn to scale, outer longitudinal layer not included)

The Neural Control of the Lower Urinary Tract

Control of the lower urinary tract is achieved through both branches of the autonomic nervous system (sympathetic and parasympathetic), and the somatomotor branch for the rhabdosphincter. Excellent in depth reviews of this topic may be found in Fowler et al. [1] and de Groat et al. [7]. For the purposes of this chapter, the following brief description should suffice.

During the storagephaseof the micturition cycle, active contraction of urethral circumferential smooth muscle and active relaxation of bladder smooth muscle are achieved via sympathetic stimulation of alpha-adrenergic and beta-adrenergic receptors, respectively, via the hypogastric nerves. In this case, the same neurotransmitter, norepinephrine, results in different effects because of regional differences in receptor subtype expression. Also during the storage phase, active tonic contraction of the rhabdosphincter is achieved by special motoneurons residing in Onuf's nucleus in the sacral spinal cord whose axons course through the pudendal nerve. These neurons are activated by a bladder-to-rhabdosphincter reflex and this reflex is important in maintain continence.

For the most part, bladder filling is not sensed at the conscious level, and these storage reflexes are governed by afferent input from the bladder at the level of the spinal cord. As filling approaches bladder capacity, and therefore approaches triggering of reflex micturition, afferent input from the bladder becomes sensed at the conscious level and inhibition of the pontine micturition reflex center is applied together with conscious activation of the rhabdosphincter while the individual seeks an appropriate environment to void. **Once an appropriate environment is found or established, conscious inhibition of the micturition reflex is relaxed and parallel pathways of inhibition of the bladder-to-rhabdosphincter spinal reflex and excitation of the neurons innervating the lower urinary tract within the parasympathetic nucleus allows for voiding to ensue.**

Postganglionic parasympathetic neurons that innervate the bladder contain either the paired smooth muscle excitatory transmitters acetylcholine (ACh) and adenosine triphosphate (ATP), neuronal nitric oxide synthase (NO; nitric oxide relaxes smooth muscle), or all of these. The distribution of these transmitters is not compartmentalized between bladder and urethra, as one might have predicted, and regional selectivity (i.e. bladder contraction and urethral smooth muscle relaxation) is achieved by the distribution of soluble guanylate cyclase, the target in smooth muscle for NO. In this case, the urinary bladder smooth muscle does not contain soluble guanylate cyclase, while the urethral circumferential smooth muscle does. It is not the case that ACh and ATP will not contract urethral circumferential smooth muscle, but rather that NO relaxation overcomes these and many, if not all, neurotransmitter- and prostaglandin-induced contractions of this layer of smooth muscle [8, 9].

That NO release in the urethra results in relaxation of urethral circumferential smooth muscle, even in the face of maximal alpha-adrenergic-mediated contraction pairs nicely with the fact that ACh stimulation of the degree experienced during micturition is not blocked by beta-adrenergic-mediated relaxation [10]. Therefore, in the absence of mechanical obstruction (e.g. stricture, pelvic floor prolapse or detrusor sphincter dyssynergia), once triggered, a micturition reflex is ensured. Thus, it is not necessary to shut off reflex sympathetic input to the system as a parallel step, although this may, in fact, occur as an evolutionary redundancy.

The sequence of events for a true micturition event is as follows: Parallel signals descend from the pontine micturition center. One signal is inhibitory to Onuf's nucleus and stops the bladder-to-rhabdosphincter spinal continence reflex. The other signal is an excitatory signal to the parasympathetic nucleus of the sacral spinal cord, stimulates parasympathetic preganglionic neurons that project to the pelvic ganglia to stimulate, in turn, the parasympathetic postganglionic neurons. The latter neurons project to the bladder and urethra. At the bladder, they cause contraction at the dome that, due to the random fiber orientation, is directed centrally and downward. The longitudinal muscle layers at the bladder base through the proximal 1/2–2/3 of the pelvic urethra also contract, which forces the bladder neck open into a funnel and provides sufficient tension to maintain the funnel shape rather than allowing the base-proximal urethra to balloon out. At the same time, the circumferential smooth muscle of the urethra relaxes, allowing the funneling to occur easily. The net result of longitudinal smooth muscle contraction is both a shortening of the distance between the bladder base and the length of the urethra that does not include longitudinal smooth muscle (i.e. the bladder descends into the pelvic floor) and an expansion of the urethral lumen, both of which reduce resistance to flow.

While this reflex seems capable of doing the job as described once initiated, there are likely modulatory afferent inputs arising from the urethra that refine the duration of descending signal. For example, upon the initiation of the void, urine that enters the proximal urethra may provide positive feedback via chemosensitive, distension sensitive and flow sensitive urethral afferents to promote continued bladder contraction, helping to ensure full emptying. Barrington [11, 12] described three such reflexes that support urethral-to-bladder positive feedback:

- Barrington's Reflex 2: A urethra-spinobulbospinal-bladder reflex—this is a long loop reflex, originating from pudendal afferents in response to intraluminal fluid flow, seen as a positive feedback mechanism that promotes efficient voiding.
- Barrington's Reflex 4: A urethra-spinal-urethra reflex—this is a short loop reflex, originating from pudendal afferents in response to intraluminal fluid flow and causes relaxation of the rhabdosphincter.
- Barrington's Reflex 7: A urethra-spinal-bladder reflex—this is a short loop reflex, originating in parasympathetic afferents, may also contribute normally as a positive feedback mechanism to promote efficient voiding.

The presence of these urethral-to-bladder reflexes remains controversial in humans, and one must recognize that differences in findings from clinical human and preclinical animal studies may reflect testing conditions and/or true species differences. However, if one were to design a system for efficient voiding, one would likely design such a system with such feedback mechanisms in place. It is tempting, therefore, to predict that such reflex pathways would be prevalent across mammalian species, including humans.

Physical Principles in Urodynamics

Fluid Dynamics

There are three states of matter, solid, liquid and gas. Liquids and gasses are considered fluids, but have differences that are of great importance as far as understanding and performing urodynamics is concerned. Primarily, they differ in terms of compressibility. **Gasses are highly compressible, while liquids are not. Pascal's Law (a.k.a the Principle of Transmission of Fluid-Pressure) describes the difference in pressure between two elevations of fluid in a column as determined by the weight of the fluid between the elevations.**
  Pascal's Law: $\Delta P = \rho g (\Delta h)$

- ΔP = the hydrostatic pressure, or the difference in pressure at two points within a fluid column, due to the weight of the fluid
- ρ = the fluid density
- g = acceleration due to gravity
- Δh = the height of fluid above the point of measurement, or the difference in elevation between the two points within the fluid column

This is important to understand whenever one calibrates a liquid pressure recording system in terms of height of a liquid (e.g. cm H_2O or mm Hg) using the height of the meniscus of a column of liquid. Here a column can mean any closed outlet tubing with an open reservoir at the elevated end.

Pascal's Law not only applies to arbitrarily designated or physically defined elevations in a column of liquid, but also for any volume of liquids confined in a rigid space. This, therefore, means that any changes in pressure applied at any given point of the liquid are transmitted equally, instantaneously and with high fidelity throughout the continuum of the confined liquid volume.

This is not the case for gasses, which are compressible and therefore damp the pressure change and take time to attain a new steady state following applied pressure changes. **Gasses in line with a liquid pressure recording system, either by design or accident (liquid in lines not degassed) have the effect of decreasing fidelity of pressure changes and force application relationships [13], and therefore are best avoided.**

Pressure-Flow relationships are utilized to diagnose outlet obstruction and bladder contractility issues [14]. Flow is defined as the quantity of fluid that has moved past a point in a given unit of time:

$$F = Q/t = \Delta Q$$

- F = flow
- Q = quantity
- t = time
- ΔQ = rate of change of mass or volume

As liquid flows through tubes, there is resistance between the fluid and vessel wall that opposes the flow.

$$R = \Delta P / \Delta Q$$

- R = resistance
- ΔP = change in pressure
- ΔQ = flow

These principles can be utilized, with important modifications to account for the biomechanical properties of the bladder and urethra, to determine outlet resistance and bladder contractile strength. In non-living systems (flexible catheters, solid tubes), R may be considered as constant. But in living systems, such as the urethra, R is dynamic and depends on the neuromuscular systems comprising the urethral outlet complex. In order to best represent the living system during urodynamic pressure flow studies, detrusor pressure at maximum voiding flow rate ($P_{det}\ Q_{max}$) and maximum voiding flow rate (Q_{max}) are plotted against each other to produce nomograms. Regions within the nomogram that represent degrees of outlet obstruction and strengths of bladder contractility are defined from mixed groups of patients [15].

Biomechanics of the Lower Urinary Tract

Biomechanics is the application of mechanical principles to living organisms and/or their tissues. Classical mechanics involves determinations of pressure, force, flow and resistance, which we have already discussed for fluid dynamics as they pertain to urodynamic investigations. Additionally, as we are dealing with tissues, considerations of solid mechanics are also important. Solid mechanical measures include stress (intensity of internal forces), strain (deformation; change in the metric properties), stiffness (resistance of an elastic body to deformation), compliance (reciprocal of stiffness), isotropy (uniformity in all directions) and anisotropy (directionally dependent). Solid behaviors in response to applied stresses include rigidity (resistance of shape change), plasticity (permanence of deformation following removal of applied stress), elasticity and viscoelasticity (both return to undeformed state, but viscoelastic solids have damping resulting in hysteresis in the stress-strain curve).

We have already discussed that the dome of the bladder has randomly oriented fibers and the base and urethra have longitudinal and circumferential fiber layers, and thus we may further define these regions as isotropic and anisotropic, respectively.

Compliance (the inverse of stiffness) is clearly an important component of urodynamic analysis.

$$C = \Delta V / \Delta P$$

- C = compliance
- ΔV = change in volume
- ΔP = change in pressure

A highly compliant bladder changes little in pressure with increasing volume, while a low compliance bladder changes pressure more rapidly with filling volume. It is important to recognize, however, that contractile tissues have three states of activity that affect compliance due to differences in resting tension:

- **Active**—in a state of paracrine- or neurocrine-mediated contraction
- **Passive**—unstimulated by paracrine or neurocrine activators, endogenous myogenic contractile tone only (autocrine, juxtacrine < gap junctions >, pacemaker potentials)
- **Inactive**—acontractile state (active relaxation by smooth muscle relaxants), reflects the biomechanical properties of the cell walls and extracellular matrix

Compliance decreases as activity state, and therefore wall tension, increases. One can approximate wall tension in the bladder using LaPlace's Law for hollow spheres:

$$T = (P * r) / 2$$

- T = wall tension
- P = pressure
- r = radius

LaPlace's Law, however, assumes that the shape is a sphere and that the wall of the sphere is isotropic. We know that these assumptions are not true of the urinary bladder, and therefore one must understand that wall tension calculations based on LaPlace's Law are inaccurate estimates.

Stress and strain are also important considerations and have been shown to affect urodynamic readouts. For example, Coolsaet [16] describes rate and time dependency of stress effects on compliance in urinary bladders. Rapid filling (fast stress) causes both a decrease in compliance and increases the time to achieve equilibrium (the true pressure-volume relationship). Thus fill rates may have significant effects on urodynamic outcomes. In addition, the bladder appears to be viscoelastic, that is to say that the pressure-volume relationship is different for the same rates of filling and emptying (lower pressures at the same volumes during emptying when compared to filling).

Conclusions

It becomes increasingly apparent that balloon and straw models of the bladder and urethra will not provide sufficient understanding of Urodynamics. Rather, an understanding of the anatomy, physiology and biomechanical properties of the system, together with an appreciation of fluid mechanics (fluid vs. air) bring to life the data obtained by Urodynamic procedures.

References

1. Fowler CJ, Griffiths D, de Groat WC. The neural control of micturition. Nat Rev Neurosci. 2008;9(6):453–66.
2. Viana R, Batourina E, Huang H, Dressler GR, Kobayashi A, Behringer RR, Shapiro E, Hensle T, Lambert S, Mendelsohn C. The development of the bladder trigone, the center of the anti-reflux mechanism. Development. 2007;134(20):3763–9.
3. Miftahof RN, Nam HG. Biomechanics of the human urinary bladder. Berlin: Springer; 2013.
4. Tanagho EA, Smith DR. The anatomy and function of the bladder neck. Br J Urol. 1966;38(1):54–71.
5. Dass N, McMurray G, Greenland JE, Brading AF. Morphological aspects of the female pig bladder neck and urethra: quantitative analysis using computer assisted 3-dimensional reconstructions. J Urol. 2001;165(4):1294–9.
6. Elbadawi A. Comparative neuromorphology in animals. In: Torrens M, Morrison JFB, editors. The physiology of the lower urinary tract. London: Springer; 1987. p. 23–51.
7. de Groat WC, Fraser MO, Yoshiyama M, Smerin S, Tai C, Chancellor MB, Yoshimura N, Roppolo JR. Neural control of the urethra. Scand J Urol Nephrol Suppl. 2001;35(207):35–43.
8. Dokita S, Morgan WR, Wheeler MA, Yoshida M, Latifpour J, Weiss RM. NG-nitro-L-arginine inhibits non-adrenergic, non-cholinergic relaxation in rabbit urethral smooth muscle. Life Sci. 1991;48(25):2429–36.
9. Garcia-Pascual A, Costa G, Garcia-Sacristan A, Andersson KE. Relaxation of sheep urethral muscle induced by electrical stimulation of nerves: involvement of nitric oxide. Acta Physiol Scand. 1991;141(4):531–9.
10. Sadananda P, Drake MJ, Paton JF, Pickering AE. A functional analysis of the influence of β3-adrenoceptors on the rat micturition cycle. J Pharmacol Exp Ther. 2013;347(2):506–15.
11. Barrington FJF. The component reflexes of micturition in the cat. Brain. 1931;54:177–88.
12. Barrington FJF. The component reflexes of micturition in the cat. Part III. Brain. 1941;64:239–43.
13. Cooper MA, Fletter PC, Zaszczurynski PJ, Damaser MS. Comparison of air-charged and water-filled urodynamic pressure measurement catheters. Neurourol Urodyn. 2011;30(3):329–34.
14. Damaser MS, Lehman SL. Two mathematical models explain the variation in cystometrograms of obstructed urinary bladders. J Biomech. 1996;29:1615–9.
15. Nitti VW. Pressure flow urodynamic studies: the gold standard for diagnosing bladder outlet obstruction. Rev Urol. 2005;7 Suppl 6:S14–21.
16. Coolsaet B. Bladder compliance and detrusor activity during the collection phase. Neurourol Urodyn. 1985;4:263–73.

Urodynamics Equipment: What the Clinician Needs to Know to Set Up the Lab

Andrew P. Windsperger and Brian J. Flynn

Planning of a Urodynamic Service and Laboratory

The development of an active, complex urodynamics (UDS) practice requires careful planning, discussion, negotiation, and coordination among a variety of individuals including nurses, physician extenders, physicians, financial officers, medical director and Urodynamic vendors. The urodynamic director ultimately needs to decide what services (GU, GI) and specialties (Urology, Urogyencology, Colorectal Surgery) will utilize the laboratory and what level of investigation and/or therapy will be available (basic UDS, advanced UDS, video UDS (VUDS), anal manometry, biofeedback, etc).

The initial step in creating an active urodynamics service is development of a referral practice. This initially starts with performing studies within one's own practice. Typically one provider and one urotechnician are involved in the evaluation of voiding dysfunction for the practice. Overtime, the practitioner may organize and interpret UDS studies for the entire group and smaller neighboring practices. Common indications for UDS include BPH, urinary retention, urinary incontinence and neurogenic bladder dysfunction. Pediatric UDS are best performed at a Children's Hospital as there are special needs in children that are not ordinarily addressed in an adult hospital or office.

Once a decision is made on the specialties utilizing the lab and level of investigation, a decision will need to be made about space, equipment, and personnel.

A.P. Windsperger, M.D.
Department of Urology, St. Cloud Hospital, CentraCare Health, Adult and Pediatric Urology of Sartell, 2351 Connecticut Ave South, Suite #200, Sartell, MN 56377, USA
e-mail: andrew.windsperger@centracare.com

B.J. Flynn, M.D. (✉)
Department of Surgery/Urology, University of Colorado Denver, 12631 East 17th Ave., Box C319, Room L15-5602, Aurora, CO 80045, USA
e-mail: brian.flynn@ucdenver.edu

Table 1 List of major urodynamics manufacturers

Laborie	Medtronic
Medical Measurement Systems International	Cooper Surgical
Dantec Medical	NeoMedix
SRS Medical	AyMed
Status Medical Equipments	Andromeda
MediPlus	TIC Medizintechnik
The Prometheus Group	Schippers-Medizintechnik

Elaborate studies require more extensive space, equipment and personnel to optimize the study. Choices vary widely between UDS systems including those designed for stationary versus portable monitoring (Table 1). High volume centers may require more advanced urodynamic testing as opposed to a center that performs only occasional testing and thus requires less equipment. For the purposes of this chapter, the focus will be on the components necessary to develop an advanced urodynamics and/or VUDS laboratory.

It is paramount that the room and personnel are dedicated to urodynamics. Urodynamic programs are doomed to fail if the lab, institution, and/or personnel are not dedicated to the urodynamic practice. Sadly, many large institutions spend as much as $250,000 on UDS equipment only to house the equipment in an operating room, radiology, or cystoscopysuite without appointing a urodynamic director or technician. Consequently, the UDS service may perform 0–4 low quality UDS studies/month. Certainly these institutions would have been better served by referring their patients to a high volume center or to utilize the services of a mobile unit.

The UDS room should be an isolated space that remains quiet without distraction during the study, as well as protect the privacy of the patient during a sensitive and potentially embarrassing procedure. **Every effort should be made to create a testing environment that allows the patient to feel comfortable so that the most physiologically accurate and "natural" results are displayed.** If the room is remote from the urology clinic such as in a radiology suite or operating room, and the staff consists of personnel from a float pool or other departments, then the UDS program may fail due to a large amount of inconvenience for both the patient and practitioner. Therefore, if VUDS is going to be utilized it is paramount that this performed in a urology suite. Urodynamics is an intimate part of the patient's evaluation and the patient is more comfortable in a familiar, safe, and private environment. Patients generally find it uncomfortable and embarrassing to have UDS performed in congested areas by personnel that are not proficient in investigating private and intimate issues involving pelvic health. The room should also allow adequate space for the UDS equipment, UDS chair/table as well as ample space for the patient, urotechnician, and the clinician. Accessibility for patients with physical limitations and appropriate space for storage of personal assistive devices such as walkers, crutches/canes, or wheelchairs is necessary.

A discussion of setting up an Urodynamic Service would be incomplete without addressing the personnel required to perform a meaningful urodynamic evaluation. Having a trained, supportive, attentive staff is vital to obtaining UDS that will provide accurate clinical information. **The staff's proper attention to correct calibration, zeroing of equipment, placement of catheters and electrodes, and interpretation and documentation of events is vital in obtaining a quality study.** The staff, bioengineering, or UDS vendor should perform calibration of equipment regularly in order to ensure accurate measurement. The urotechnician should have a detailed understanding of catheter placement and study protocols in order to assist with any necessary troubleshooting. Typically the UDS personnel are either a physician extender, a nurse, or medical assistant trained in the performance of UDS known as a urotechnician. A physician extender is usually not required unless they plan on operating radiology equipment or interpreting the study. What is most important is that the person performing the study is well trained and proficient in UDS. The leading UDS manufacturers conduct formal training seminars, and organizations such as the Society of Urologic Nurses and Associates (SUNA) also offer continuing education opportunities (Table 2).

Preparing for a Urodynamic Study

Before the UDS appointment the patient's records should be reviewed in advance to determine if there are any special needs (lift, interpreter, etc.). The patient should arrive to their urodynamic appointment with a 3–7 day bladder log, pad weight test when applicable and a completed validated urinary questionnaire such as the UDI-6, AUA symptom score, or Kings Health. Urine analysis and pre-procedure antibiotics are never required for *basic UDS* as this is non invasive (See chapter "The Clinical Evaluation of the Patient Who Requires Urodynamics").

Correlation with clinical data is the most important part of the urodynamic study. Most urodynamic practitioners insist on performing a consultation that would include history and physical and evaluation of other objective measures before performing the urodynamic study. **The urodynamic study is unlike a radiologic study that may be performed in isolation remote from the practitioner. Rather, the urodynamicist should interact with the patient regularly and have a report**

Table 2 Necessary items for creating a friendly atmosphere that creates a private environment for the patient

1. A dedicated bathroom and changing facilities within a secure area
2. A dedicated UDS procedure room with a door lock and curtains around the entrance and exit to the room
3. Control over the flow of personnel into and out of the room
4. Dedicated, well-trained UDS personnel

with the patient to fully understand the goals of the study in order to properly design the study, make a diagnosis and formulate a treatment plan.

Types of Urodynamic Investigation

In this section we will review the typical setting in which each of UDS modalities are best utilized. We will discuss the room, equipment and personnel needed. We will comment on the cost, advantages and disadvantages of each modality and how to best incorporate each into your practice.

The urodynamic equipment and organization of an urodynamic unit for evaluation of urinary dysfunction varies based on the level of investigation. Each level of urodynamics investigation requires different equipment, room design and personnel. There are three sections of investigation:

- **Basic Urodynamics**: this would include measurement of simple uroflow (Q), measurement of post void residual (PVR) and single channel cystometry
- **Advanced Urodynamics (UDS)**: this would include a multi-channel study along with patch EMG electrodes
- **VideoUrodynamics**: would include all components of advanced urodynamics with the addition of fluoroscopy fluro-urodynamics (FUDS) or more commonly video urodynamics (VUDS)

Basicurodynamics can be performed in almost any size urology or urogynecology office/clinic and even in some primary care, neurology, spine and rehabilitation clinics. A **bladder scanner** is a non-invasive method that uses ultrasound to measure pos-void residual. It is widely available in hospital emergency rooms, recovery rooms, and medical-surgical wards. The space required for basic urodynamics is minimal, and in most instances can be wall-mounted in a bathroom (Fig. 1). The technical equipment is simple and inexpensive and accessible to most office settings. The personal required would be the existing medical assistant with supervision of a physician or physician extender.

Uroflowometry Uroflowometry is another non-invasive part of the urodynamic process that measures the flow rate. Flow rates are generally reported in milliliters per second (mL/s), though measurements generally are recorded in either kilograms per second (kg/s) or cubic meters per second (m^3/s). Most uroflowometers are calibrated for water (1 g/mL) that allows for calculations that operate under the assumption that the mass of the fluid in grams equals the volume in milliliters. This becomes important when using instillation agents other than water, such as contrast medium for video studies, as the true density of the fluid may alter the actual flow rate compared to the calculated, reported flow rate. In the case of a denser fluid, such as contrast medium, this would lead to an artificially elevated calculated flow rate relative to the actual flow rate. Detailed calibration can assist with limiting any potential discordance between calculated and actual flow rates. Additional

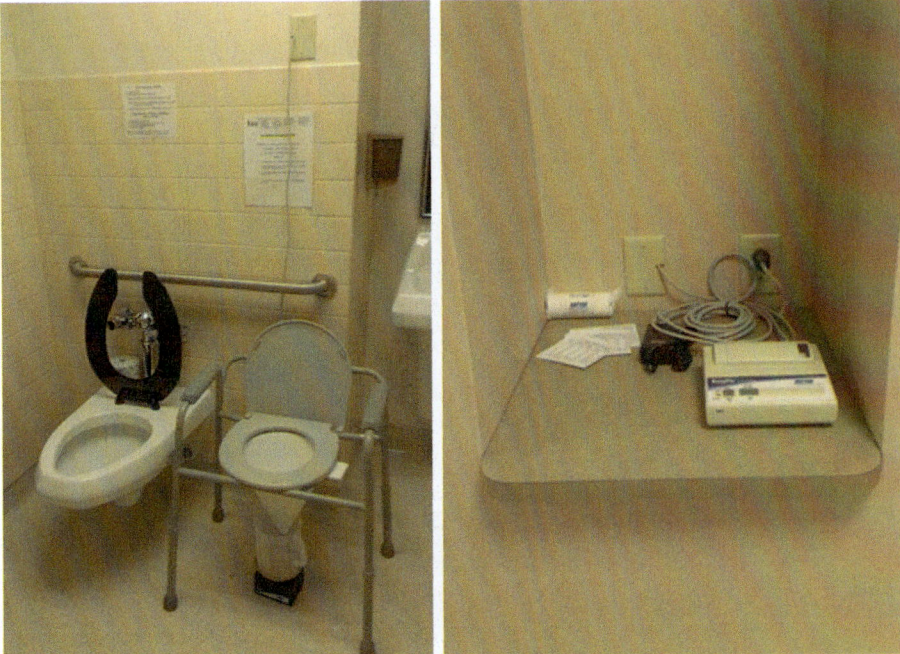

Fig. 1 Demonstrates a non-invasive uroflow with wall-mounted unit and output/printer

calibration standards per ICS guidelines allow for expected delays between initiation of voiding and initiation of the study, though advancements in automation have improved detection of study initiation in new uroflowometers [1].

The majority of uroflowometers available are of a gravity-based design. Voided fluid is measured either by weight or by hydrostatic pressure, and a value is derived that is proportional to the mass of fluid collected. Rotating disk flowmeters involve a rotating disk that continues at a constant rate; voided fluid is directed onto the disk, and the power required to keep the disk rotating at its constant is measured. This is proportional to the mass flow rate of the fluid. Finally, electronic dipstick flowmeters measure the electrical capacitance of a dipstick placed within the collection chamber. The flow rate is derived from the output signal of the device, which is proportional to the total volume accumulated within the chamber [2].

Automation and technological integration has assisted in measurement of uroflowometry, not only in attempting to improve the automated reporting of initiated voiding, but also in providing improved connectivity options for data reporting. Many uroflowometers are now equipped with wireless or Bluetooth reporting options that communicate directly with electronic records and office computer interfaces. A home smart phone application is also available that attempts to assist patients in estimation of their flow rates based upon voided volume/time.

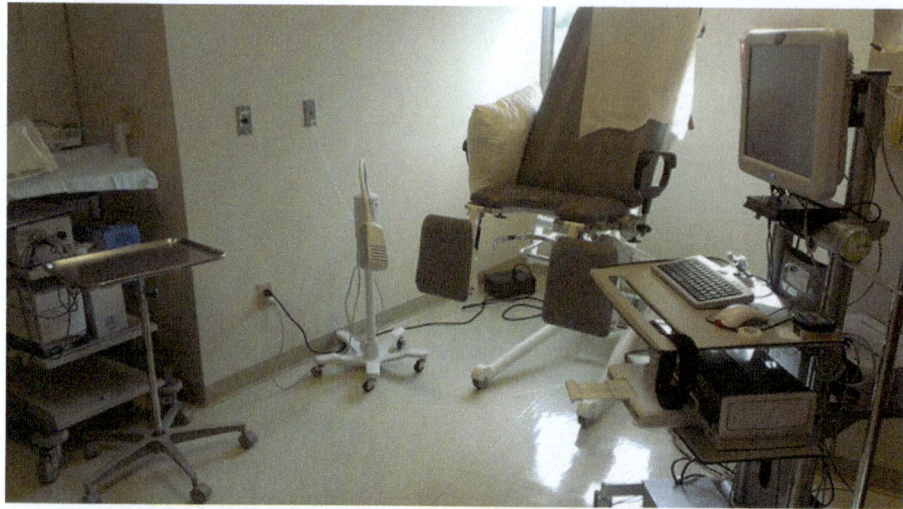
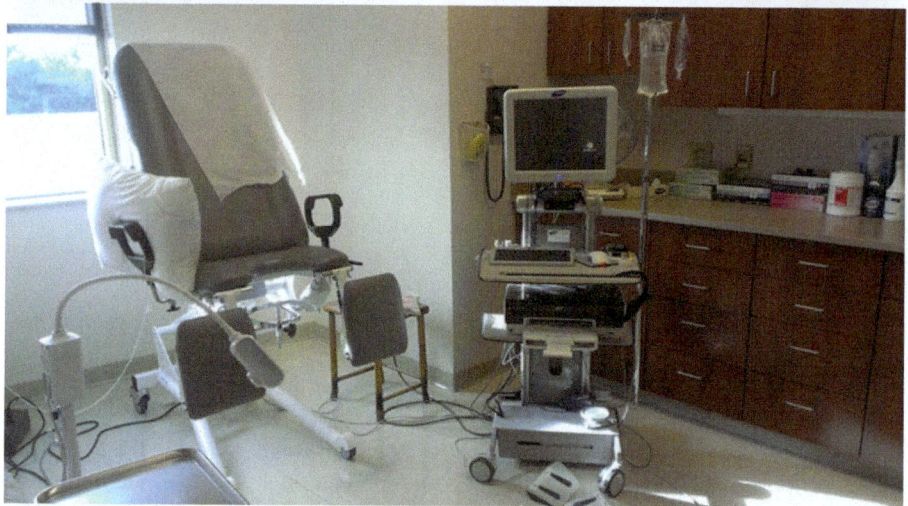

Fig. 2 Example of an advanced urodynamics

Advancedurodynamics is usually performed by medium-large Urology or Urogynecology offices or clinics that usually consist of more than five physicians and at least that many support staff members. In most large offices, tertiary care centers, and teaching hospitals there is a large (2–3× size of an ordinary exam room) room dedicated to only Urodynamics (Fig. 2). The table and equipment is left in place and the room is ideally utilized for 8–10 h/5 days/week. The equipment is considerably more expensive than basic equipment and the price is quite variable depending on the hardware, monitor, networking, and ability to integrate with electronic health records. Typically there are 2–4 urotechnicians (one technician/study) that staff the laboratory.

Cystometrogam (CMG) In 2002, the International Continence Society described a set of minimum standards for the equipment used to conduct advanced UDS. These include: (1) three channels, two for pressure and one for flow, (2) a computerized display/monitor, (3) secure storage of the recorded pressures (abdominal, vesical, detrusor), (4) flow measurements as tracings versus time. The infused volume must be recorded graphically and/or numerically. There must be a method for event annotation to mark information about sensation and additional comments during the study. All measured and derived signals are to be displayed continuously over time according to ICS standards, with a recommended order of Pabd (abdominal pressure), Pves (vesical pressure), Pdet (detrusor pressure), and flow (Q). The system software must ensure that information for pressures up to 250 cm H_2O and flow rates up to 50 mL/s are recorded (see Table 3; additional minimal standards are listed in Fig. 1) [1].

Electromyography (EMG) Multiple options also exist for the recording of electromyography during the urodynamic evaluation. Invasive and non-invasive options are available, and the use of each should be determined by the specific question that needs to be answered by the study. Non-invasive options such as skin patch electrodes allow for both patient comfort and mobility, but only offer a global kinesiologic view of muscle coordination. If a more specific evaluation is necessary, Invasive options such as needle electrodes, wire electrodes, monopolar electrodes,

Table 3 CMG software requirements

Accuracy	±1 cm H_2O for pressure
	±5 % of the full scale for flow
Detection ranges	0–250 cm H_2O for pressure
	0–50 mL/s for flow
	0–1000 mL for volume
Time constant	0.75 s
Software	No loss of data for pressures up to 250 cm H_2O and flow up to 50 mL/s
Frequency	Analog/digital frequency of 10 Hz per channel
	20 kHz minimum may be needed for EMG
Printout	Line resolution better than 0.10 mm
Maximum deflection	
Pressure	200 cm H_2O
Flow	50 mL/s
Volume	1000 mL
Minimum scaling	
Pressure	50 cm H_2O per cm
Flow	10 mL/s per cm
Time axis	1 min/cm or 5 s/mm for filling
	2 s/mm for voiding

or concentric electrodes offer views of individual motor units. However, needle EMG may be uncomfortable for patients and limits their mobility during the study. Moreover, needle EMG monitoring requires expertise that most technicians and physicians do not have thereby limiting its clinical application.

Video urodynamics (VUDS) also known as Fluroscopic urodynamics (FUDS) is performed in approximately 5 % of UDS settings and is reserved for large Urology Centers (10 or more physicians), Hospital, and University-based UDS labs. This is the highest level of investigation as fluoroscopy is conveniently added to advanced urodynamics. The video portion provides simultaneous structural and anatomic data to complex CMG and Pressure/Flow studies. This is sometimes considered the gold standard in urodynamics. This allows a comprehensive interactive elaborate study of voiding dysfunction. Many clinical answers can be achieved in a single study. For example, simultaneous pressure flow measurement with voiding cystourethrogram can detect not only the obstruction, but also demonstrate the shape and contour of the bladder as well as screen for vesicoureteral reflux.

In most centers, there is a very large (4× the size of an ordinary exam room) room dedicated to only Video-Urodynamics (Fig. 3). The cost of this room includes the cost of advanced equipment, with additional expense of software required to integrate the UDS with fluoroscopy in a single display and report, the cost of an x-ray compatible table and the cost of a C-arm fluoroscopy. A fixed urology

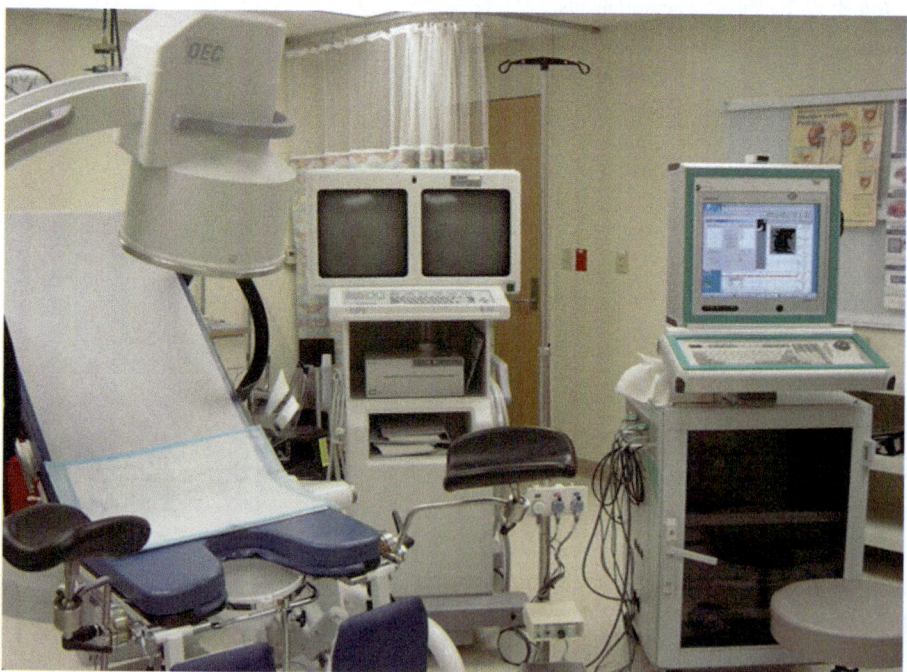

Fig. 3 Example of advanced urodynamics with videourodynamic capabilities

table is only useful for filling cystogram and does not allow video of a patient in a seated position during micturition. The support staff would include the urotechnicians needed for advanced UDS as well as additional cost of a radiology technician. The price is likely prohibitive for most small centers. There is usually a physician in the practice that has specialized in Female Pelvic Medicine or Neurourology with an active practice in bladder and pelvic health. The equipment and personnel for a VUDS laboratory is more extensive, and hence expensive, in this setting.

A lead-lined room is not required in most settings if the amount of radiation from that room is minimal. A VUDS room with a C-arm where fluoroscopic exams are performed infrequently does not require lead-lining. Even in a busy clinic that performs four or more cases per day, the total fluoroscopy time would total approximately 2 min or less. This is a minimal amount of time, and therefore the requirement for a lead lines room is not necessary unless the room is next to a sensitive population such as infants.

Advanced UDS vs VUDS Those who are not in favor of VUDS would argue that VUDS is an expensive way of obtaining information that can be obtained equally well by combining urodynamics with other studies, such as cystoscopy or voiding cystourethrography. This would require a separate catheterization of course and possibly two separate appointments, one to urology and one to radiology. However, the same proponents argue that the room size and the need for a C-arm and an x-ray table cannot be justified in most centers. There are a number of political and organizational challenges in hospital and university-based units that make the organization of a video urodynamic suite complicated. The lack of reimbursement to urologists for interpretation of radiologic studies (VCUG) and the lack of reimbursement to the facility for fluoroscopy and contrast medium have created a crisis in many UDS centers. That is, it is hard to justify the expense of the additional equipment and personnel for VUDS without any additional reimbursement to the practice or hospital. This dilemma is further amplified by the significant cuts in reimbursement to basic and advanced UDS.

At the University of Colorado we can perform 6–8 advanced urodynamic studies/day in non-neurogenic ambulatory patients. However, if VUDS is utilized we can perform only four studies/day even with an additional UDS technician. The demand of a busy urodynamic laboratory often overwhelms the urodynamic slots if VUDS is employed without additional room and personnel. For these reasons, along with the increased time required to perform VUDS, there has been a significant decrease in the utilization of VUDS in the last 5–10 years in the United States. If VUDS is not available, it is appropriate to perform advanced UDS and then have the patient evaluated in radiology with voiding cystourethrogram (VCUG). This of course requires more than one urethral catheterization which is an inconvenience to some patients. However, many of the patients that require VUDS are neurogenic bladder patients on self-catheterization. One possible compromise in a large practice setting would be to: (1) equip multiple bathrooms for basic UDS for simple uroflow and measurement of post void residual, (2) have a UDS room equipped for advanced studies, (3) have a separate room dedicated to VUDS.

Computerized Urodynamics, Data Processing and Data Storage

In today's digital world, analog information is becoming obsolete. **Virtually all urodynamic equipment will convert analoginformationinto an output that is user friendly, easily displayed, and shared either electronically or by a paper report**. The days of printing out urodynamic analog tracings on scrolling paper and compiling a hand written 'fill-in-the-blank report' have gone into the archives. Although urodynamic information is still created in an analog signal that contains information using non-quantized variations in frequency and amplitude, the information is then converted into a continuous digital signal using an analog-to-digital converter on the PC hard drive. The digital signal is a physical signal that is a representation of a sequence of discrete values, known as a digitized analog signal. This information then may be displayed on a high definition computer monitor and recorded on the hard drive and printed out for as a formal report. The design of the urodynamic report is up to the practitioner. Many vendors provide generic reports that have simple templates that can be used and shared amongst practitioners. Other urodynamic practitioners prefer to personalize their reports including not only urodynamic reports but also clinical information. The entire study may be shown on a single piece of paper with a compressed tracing, event summary, report and representative video pictures.

Data Recording and documentation is vital in the urodynamic process. The study is typically saved on the hard drive of the urodynamic computer. The computer is usually connected to a color printer as this allows an easy method of sharing studies with patients and referring doctors. In some centers the urodynamic computer interfaces with the electronic medical (EMR) record to allow storage into a commonly shared EMR in large hospital settings. However, there continues to be a number of technical, proprietary and software issues that make sharing information electronically difficult. Consequently, the most common form of UDS data storage is on-site hard drive, or paper printed out. The urodynamics study should be archived and available for future review and comparison to prior studies. A large data bank of urodynamic studies can usually be compiled if a hard drive is suitable (500 GB–1 TB hard drive). **We recommend having a reproducible and reliable filing system so studies can be retrieved either by name, date, or by medical record number.** UDS information is easily transferred to external devices such as an external hard drive, USB, zip drive, or CD. However, in order to display and review the UDS information recorded on an external device the computer, tablet, or hand held device, the device must have a copy of the urodynamic software used to create the study.

We highly recommend that the UDS-computer be connected to the Internet via a hard-wired Ethernet cord. This allows for remote calibration, remote troubleshooting, and remote installation of updated software. Additionally, remote access and control of the UDS computer may be necessary when involved in a clinical trial that requires a uniform urodynamic study and template that can be shared amongst collaborators.

Conclusions

It is our opinion that basic UDS is required for 100 % of urology practices. Advanced urodynamics would be necessary for the majority (70 %) of practices especially those that commonly see complex patients from other specialists. If the practice is too small to afford the cost, space, or personnel for this service, a mobile vendor may be considered to meet the needs of the practice. Dependent on the practice setting and patient characteristics we estimate video urodynamics is necessary in only 5–20 % of urodynamics studies.

The urodynamic results should never trump the clinical picture; rather, the interpretation of the UDS study should correlate directly with the patient's symptoms. If faced with a discrepancy such as a contradiction between the history and physical versus the urodynamic study, it is important to rely more on the clinical picture. A study may be repeated in effort to corroborate results. If the results don't make sense, then one needs to repeat the study or repeat the history. Erroneous data and misinterpretation of urodynamics can lead to serious clinical consequences such as misdiagnosis. Finally, urodynamic studies should not be painful for the patient, the technician, or the practitioner. Rather, it should be a valuable piece of the patient's record used to guide medical and surgical therapy and help predict which patients may develop upper urinary tract deterioration as a result of untreated bladder dysfunction.

References

1. Schaefer W, Abrams P, Liao L, et al. Good urodynamic practices: uroflowometry, filling cystometry, and pressure-flow studies. Neurourol Urodyn. 2002;21:261–74.
2. Wein A, editor. Campbell-Walsh urology—Ch 62: Urodynamic and video-urodynamic testing of the lower urinary tract. 10th ed. Maryland Heights, MO: WB Saunders; 2011.

The Clinical Evaluation of the Patient Who Requires Urodynamics

Maria Voznesensky and R. Clay McDonough III

Introduction

Urodynamic testing is a useful diagnostic tool for the evaluation of the patient with lower urinary tract dysfunction. **Before proceeding with urodynamics testing, the clinician should perform a thorough diagnostic evaluation in order to determine both the necessity of testing as well as the appropriate urodynamic study.** This chapter will discuss the pre-urodynamic workup, current guidelines for the use of urodynamics, and patient preparation and education.

History

As with any patient, a complete history is necessary to obtain a clear understanding of the patient's complaints. The physician should inquire about the nature of the patient's symptoms (i.e., urgency, frequency, urge and/or stress incontinence, bladder pain, and dysuria), severity and duration of symptoms, degree of bother associated with the complaints, any previous therapies that have been attempted, and other relevant medical comorbidities.

Neurologic diseasecan often have an impact on lower urinary tract function, and it is important to review both known neurologic diagnoses as well as symptoms that would be associated with neurologic disorders. Additional important information includes the presence of dyspareunia, effect of symptoms on sexual function, history of pelvic radiation therapy, hematuria, and any prior genitourinary or gynecological surgeries. In female patients, a complete obstetric and menstrual history

M. Voznesensky, M.D. • R.C. McDonough III, M.D. (✉)
Department of Urology, Maine Medical Center, 100 Brickhill Ave.,
South Portland, ME 04106, USA
e-mail: voz.maria@gmail.com; mcurodoc@gmail.com

should be obtained to include parity and mode of all deliveries. All medications should be reviewed as they could potentially contribute to the patient's condition.

Standardized validated questionnaires exist to aid the clinician in evaluating symptoms, degree of bother, and quality of life [1]. Two widely used symptoms tools are the Urogenital Distress Inventory Short Form (UDI-6) and the International Consultation of Incontinence Questionnaire Short Form on Urinary Incontinence (ICIQ-UI). Additionally, the American Urologic Association Symptom Score (AUASS) and International Prostate Severity Score (I-PSS) may be extremely useful in the pre-study evaluation of patients with any type of lower urinary tract symptoms.

Physical Examination

Physical examination may identify specific findings which could contribute to or cause the symptoms of interest. Examples include pelvic prolapse, urethral diverticulum, or an abdominal/pelvic mass. Additionally, findings on exam may change one's approach to clinical management. Special care or change in management may be required for patients with compromised mobility/dexterity or compromised mental status.

A complete examination should include assessment of the abdomen, back, genitalia, perineum, rectum, and neurologic system. Specifically, one should evaluate general mental status, body mass index, physical dexterity and mobility, abnormal gait, and extremity weakness. The abdomen and flank should be examined for masses, bladder distention, and relevant surgical scars.

Both a speculum and digital exam (bimanual and anorectal) should be performed in female patients. During speculum examination, a stress test can be performed to look for stress urinary incontinence. Degree of pelvic prolapse can be assessed using the Pelvic Organ Prolapse Quantification System (POP-Q). Pelvic muscle tone and the presence of any pelvic mass should be noted. In men, the penis, scrotum, and testes should be inspected. A rectal exam will reveal resting anal tone as well as allow for examination of the prostate. Prostate exam should include evaluation for mass, enlargement, and tenderness. In both sexes, the skin of the genitalia and perineum should be examined for evidence of breakdown or infection which may result from their complaint (Table 1).

Laboratory Evaluation

Urinalysis (UA) is a useful screening and diagnostic tool that provides rapid results in the office setting. **A simple UA can be used to rule out urinary tract infection, screen for microscopic hematuria, and identify causes of secondary incontinence such as glucosuria, pyuria, and proteinuria.** Urine culture is also helpful

Table 1 Physical examination

Both	Male	Female
General mental status		
Body mass index		
Dexterity and mobility		
Abdomen, flank		
Skin		
Perineum		
Genitals	Penis	Vaginal half-speculum exam
	Scrotum	Bimanual pelvic and anorectal
	Testicles	Stress test for incontinence
	Hernia	Urethral diverticulum
	Digital rectal exam	Pelvic mass
		Pelvic muscle tone

in the diagnosis of urinary tract infection. Microscopic hematuria should not be ignored in this patient population, as urinary tract malignancy may present as new onset urinary urgency/frequency or urge incontinence—a full urologic hematuria workup may be appropriate. At times, it can be difficult in some female patients to provide a specimen that does not exhibit vaginal contamination (as evidenced by the presence of vaginal squamous epithelial cells). This can be encountered in patients with pelvic organ prolapse, obesity, and in patients who may have limited coordination. In this circumstance, it is often helpful to obtain a sample via catheterization.

The basic metabolic panel (BMP) is often used as a surrogate for renal function assessment. Although not necessary in all patients, biochemical tests for renal function are recommended in patients with urinary incontinence and known or high probability renal impairment. Some of the neurogenic bladder population is at risk for renal deterioration, and routine BMP is useful for ongoing surveillance of the upper urinary tract.

Voiding Diary

Patients should complete a voiding diary to objectively assess fluid intake, voided volume, episodes of incontinence, and voiding frequency as well as functional capacity avoiding, maximal bladder capacity, and nocturia. These diaries may document intake and voiding behavior which may be useful for patient education and for documenting both baseline symptoms and treatment efficacy. Table 2 is an example of the voiding diary used at our institution. The voiding diary has multiple advantages. It is an inexpensive test that involves the patient in their treatment program. It is also a reasonable substitute for cystometry—the largest voided volume on the voiding diary has been demonstrated to correlate with the

Table 2 Example voiding diary

Time	Amount voided (in cc's or ounces)	Leak volume 1 = drops/damp 2 = wet- 3 = bladder emptied	Activity during leak	Urge? Yes/No	Fluid intake (amount in ounces/type)

patient's cystometric capacity [2]. The diary objectively determines a reasonable voiding interval to begin a program of bladder training and establishes a way to measure change with therapy [3]. In addition to the above advantages, clinicians may use the diary to guide the conduct of urodynamics by using information such as the average voided volume to establish more physiologic bladder capacities at which certain tests such as leak point pressures are evaluated.

Pad Weight Testing

Pad weight testing helps to objectively quantify the amount of urine lost during incontinent episodes. Several methods of performing this test have been documented. Traditionally, gynecological literature describes instilling 250 mL of saline into the bladder, followed by asking the patient to complete a series of activities over 60 min (walking, climbing stairs, coughing, etc.) while wearing a pad. If the weight of the pad increases by 2–3 g over the hour, the test is considered positive.

Alternatively, patients are asked to wear pads over varying intervals of time (ranging from 1 to 72 h) and to collect and return the used pads to the physician. These pads are then weighed by the clinic and total urine volume lost is calculated, using a dry pad as baseline. Greater than 8 g of urine loss over 24 h with this method is considered a positive test.

Current research shows that the 1-h pad test has poor predictive value in the diagnosis of female urinary incontinence when compared to stress test and urine leakage [4–6]. Simply asking a woman if she is continent was as effective as performing the pad test and correlated more strongly with the patient quality of life. While useful for academic purposes and clinical trials, the 1 h pad test is tedious and inconvenient for the patient and often has poor compliance [7]. The Fourth International Consultation on Incontinence (ICI) Committee did not recommend pad tests as part of the initial evaluation in the incontinent patient [8].

Cystoscopy

Although not indicated in all patients, direct visualization of the lower urinary tract may be of some benefit to rule out urethral and bladder pathology. If justified by the history and physical, cystoscopy can help diagnose a number of conditions that may influence or cause the patients symptoms. Specific examples include urethral stricture, inflammation, urethral or bladder diverticula, anatomic defects, and foreign bodies. **In patients with microscopic or macroscopic hematuria and irritative symptoms, one must rule out malignancy as a cause prior to treatment. Cystoscopy is an essential component of the hematuria workup** [9].

In men with incontinence after radical prostatectomy (both before and after treatment), cystoscopy is vital to evaluation of the urethra when considering surgical intervention. **Cystoscopy provides valuable information about urethral sphincter function, can evaluate coaptation of the urethral mucosa with a previously placed artificialurinarysphincter, and can demonstrateurethraltissue atrophy if present.**

Other Ancillary Studies

The volume of urine left in the bladder following voiding is termed the postvoid residual (PVR)and should be evaluated in all incontinent patients [10]. The PVR evaluates the bladder's ability to empty. Knowing the patient has an elevated PVR can be helpful in diagnosing overflow incontinence. It also establishes a baseline for the patient, as both medical and surgical therapy may cause this to worsen. PVR measurement may not be necessary for uncomplicated patients if treatment is limited only to behavioral therapy.

Imaging studies are not required for most patients. However, in patients with hematuria, upper tract imaging is required to ensure the clinician does not miss a potentially harmful cause such as urothelial cancer or calculus disease [9]. In male patients in whom there is a high suspicion of urethral stricture, the clinician should obtain a retrograde urethrogram to both diagnose and define the severity of disease.

Current Recommendations from Guidelines on Indications for Urodynamics

Although urodynamic testing is a useful diagnostic tool for evaluating patients with lower urinary tract dysfunction, some patients may not need the full spectrum of tests available. In fact, some patients may not require urodynamic testing at all after the clinical evaluation is complete. Multiple societies have published recommendations regarding the use of urodynamics. The following recommendations are a synthesis of the published guidelines from the American Urological Association, the National Institute for Health and Clinical Excellence, the International Continence Society, the American Urogynecologic Society, and the Urinary Incontinence Treatment Network [11–16].

Urodynamics not necessary—**Urodynamic studies are optional in uncomplicated patients with stress incontinence. In addition, they are not necessary when starting a conservative treatment program.** Patients with neurogenic bladder who are at low risk of renal complications (such as most patients with multiple sclerosis), do not need to be routinely offered urodynamic testing.

Helpful—Preoperative studies can assist to counsel patients and set realistic expectations prior to surgery. **Urodynamic studies can be helpful in patients where the diagnosis remains uncertain after the initial clinical workup. It is also useful when the patient's symptoms do not correlate with objective findings. Additional situations where urodynamics are helpful include patients with mixed symptoms or who have failed prior therapies.** This includes patients with prior incontinence surgeries or prior exposure to radiation therapy. Finally, postoperative urodynamic studies can provide a useful basis for comparison to preoperative status in the event of a less than ideal treatment outcome.

Necessary—**UDS should be strongly considered prior to any invasive, potentially morbid, or irreversible procedure for stress incontinence, pelvic organ prolapse, orlower urinary tract symptoms. Clinicians shouldperformpressure flow studies in men when it is important to definitively determine if outlet obstruction is present with lower urinary tract symptoms. Lastly, urodynamics should be utilized to establish a baseline for patients withneurogenic bladder dysfunctionwho will require long term urologic management.** Voiding symptoms in this patient population can change over time; urodynamics allows for objective analysis and assists in directing therapy to prevent damage to the upper urinary tracts. Neurogenic bladder patients at high risk who should be considered for this include those with spina bifida, spinal cord injury, myelomeningocele, and anorectal abnormalities (Table 3).

Table 3 Recommendation for the use of UDS

Not necessary	Helpful	Necessary
Uncomplicated stress incontinence	Counseling, setting expectations prior to surgery	Prior to invasive, morbid, or irreversible procedures
Starting a conservative treatment program	Diagnosis remains uncertain after Hx, PE	In men, when it is important to determine if obstruction is present with LUTS
Patients at low risk of renal complications	Symptoms don't correlate with physical exam	Establish a baseline for patients with neurogenic bladder dysfunction
	Mixed symptomology	
	Failed prior therapies	
	Prior incontinence surgeries, or radiation	
	Basis for comparison in the event of a less-than-ideal surgical outcome	

Patient Preparation and Education

Patient preparation for urodynamic testing is essential, contributing to both the efficiency and usefulness of the test as well as to patient comfort. **Although typically well tolerated, urodynamics can generate feelings of anxiety, discomfort, and embarrassment; all of which may drastically effect the outcomes of the testing.** Prior to proceeding, all patient questions should be answered thoroughly. At our institution, patients also receive standard directions (Table 4) instructing them as to the following:

- Do not fast.
- Take regularly scheduled home medications.
- Arrive with a full bladder
- A urinalysis will be checked. If infected, the test will be rescheduled.
- Expect mild dysuria, hematuria, and/or increased bladder sensitivity for approximately 24 h after testing

At the time of procedure, informed consent should be signed and a final "time out" performed in accordance with institutional standards. Finally, patients with neurogenic bowels may need to be instructed to have a bowel cleanout the night before the procedure.

Periprocedural Antibiotic Treatment and Guidelines

For the average individual, urodynamics is minimally traumatic and has a low risk of causing urinary tract infections. Several randomized controlled trials demonstrate no reduction of infection rates with prophylaxis [17–19]. **The American**

Table 4 Patient instructions for urodynamic testing

You have been scheduled for a test called Urodynamic Testing (UDS). During this series of tests, your bladder will be evaluated for a variety of conditions.
When you arrive, you will be asked to empty your bladder on a special commode. It is important that you come with a comfortably full bladder and do not empty until you are asked to do so.
To start the examination, lidocaine jelly will be inserted into your urethra to numb it. A small catheter will be passed into your bladder and another catheter placed in your vagina (females) or rectum (males). Your bladder will be slowly filled with sterile water through this catheter and you will be asked to identify your sensation at different levels of fullness until you cannot hold any more of the water.
When you are completely full, you will be asked to urinate in order to assess how well your bladder contracts. The catheter may also be repositioned to evaluate the strength of your urethra.
Rarely, this test can cause a complication or problem. Less than 1 % of people will develop a bladder infection. Temporary irritation, burning with urination or a little blood in the urine is common and generally lasts only a few hours after the test.

Your preparation for the test is important:
Please do not apply lotions, powders or sprays to the pelvic area on the day of your test.
Arrive 10–15 min prior to your appointment.
Come with a comfortably full bladder and do not void until instructed to do so. (This does not apply if you have a Foley catheter or you have leakage of urine that cannot be controlled.)
If you have been asked to fill out a voiding diary in advance, bring this with you to the appointment.
You may be asked to stop medications that affect your bladder such as oxybutynin. Ask the doctor or nurse if you are not sure.

Urological Association antimicrobial prophylaxis guidelines state that antibiotic prophylaxis before urodynamics is indicated only in patients with specific risk factors [20]. These include advanced age, anatomic anomalies, poor nutrition, smoking, chronic corticosteroid use, immunodeficiency, externalized catheters, colonized materials, coexistent infection, and prolonged hospitalization. If antibiotics are used prophylactically, recommended drugs include oral fluoroquinolones or trimethroprim-sulfamethoxazole. However, the clinician should make use of local institutional antibiograms and consider patient allergies when selecting appropriate coverage.

Conclusion

Urodynamics is an important tool for the clinician who treats lower urinary tract dysfunction. **However, this testing cannot be used in isolation and does require appropriate clinical workup prior to proceeding.** With proper history, physical, and ancillary studies, the clinician can effectively select and conduct urodynamic studies to better answer clinical questions while best serving their patients.

References

1. van de Vaart H, Falconer C, Quail D, et al. Patient reported outcomes tools in an observational study of female stress urinary incontinence. Neurourol Urodyn. 2010;29(3):348–53.
2. Diokno AC, Wells TJ, Brink CA. Comparison of self-reported voided volume with cystometric bladder capacity. J Urol. 1987;137(4):698–700.
3. Hsieh CH, Chang ST, Hsieh CJ, et al. Treatment of interstitial cystitis with hydrodistention and bladder training. Int Urogynecol J Pelvic Floor Dysfunct. 2008;19(10):1379–84.
4. Abdel-fattah M, Barrington JW, Youssef M. The standard 1-hour pad test: does it have any value in clinical practice? Eur Urol. 2004;46(3):377–80.
5. Costantini E, Lazzeri M, Bini V, et al. Sensitivity and specificity of one-hour pad test as a predictive value for female urinary incontinence. Urol Int. 2008;81(2):153–9.
6. Dylewski DA, Jamison MG, Borawski KM, et al. A statistical comparison of pad numbers versus pad weights in the quantification of urinary incontinence. Neurourol Urodyn. 2007;26(1):3–7.
7. Groutz A, Blaivas JG, Chaikin DC, et al. Noninvasive outcome measures of urinary incontinence and lower urinary tract symptoms: a multicenter study of micturition diary and pad tests. J Urol. 2000;164(3 Pt 1):698–701.
8. Abrams P, Andersson KE, Birder L, et al. Fourth International Consultation on Incontinence Recommendations of the International Scientific Committee: Evaluation and treatment of urinary incontinence, pelvic organ prolapse, and fecal incontinence. Neurourol Urodyn. 2010;29(1):213–40.
9. Davis R, Jones JS, Barocas DA, et al. Diagnosis, evaluation and follow-up of asymptomatic microhematuria (AMH) in adults: AUA guideline. J Urol. 2012;188(6 Suppl):2473–81.
10. Gormley EA. Evaluation of the patient with incontinence. Can J Urol. 2007;14 Suppl 1:58–62.
11. Collins CW, Winters JC. AUA/SUFU adult urodynamics guideline: a clinical review. Urol Clin North Am. 2014;41(3):353–62.
12. Smith A, Bevan D, Douglas HR, et al. Management of urinary incontinence in women: summary of updated NICE guidance. BMJ. 2013;347:f5170.
13. Swain S, Hughes R, Perry M, et al. Management of lower urinary tract dysfunction in neurological disease: summary of NICE guidance. BMJ. 2012;345:e5074. doi:10.1136/bmj.e5074.
14. Gammie A, Clarkson B, Constantinou C, et al. International Continence Society guidelines on urodynamic equipment performance. Neurourol Urodyn. 2014;33(4):370–9.
15. Winters JC, Dmochowski RR, Goldman HB, et al. Urodynamic studies in adults: AUA/SUFU guideline. J Urol. 2012;188(6 Suppl):2464–72.
16. Nager CW, Brubaker L, Litman HJ, et al. A randomized trial of urodynamic testing before stress-incontinence surgery. N Engl J Med. 2012;366(21):1987–97.
17. Latthe PM, Foon R, Toozs-Hobson P. Prophylactic antibiotics in urodynamics: a systematic review of effectiveness and safety. Neurourol Urodyn. 2008;27(3):167–73.
18. Foon R, Toozs-Hobson P, Latthe P. Prophylactic antibiotics to reduce the risk of urinary tract infections after urodynamic studies. Cochrane Database Syst Rev. 2012;10, CD008224.
19. Böthig R, Fiebag K, Thietje R, et al. Morbidity of urinary tract infection after urodynamic examination of hospitalized SCI patients: the impact of bladder management. Spinal Cord. 2013;51(1):70–3.
20. Wolf Jr JS, Bennett CJ, Dmochowski RR, et al. Best practice policy statement on urologic surgery antimicrobial prophylaxis. J Urol. 2008;179(4):1379–90.

Noninvasive Urodynamics

Oscar Alfonso Storme and Kurt Anthony McCammon

Introduction

Urodynamics, the study of the lower urinary tract function, is designed to reproduce the lower urinary tract symptoms the patient experiences under controlled and measurable conditions for the analysis of function and dysfunction to identify the cause of symptoms [1]. The procedure provides the clinician with the necessary information to systematically approach the patient's diagnosis and choose the optimal treatment. UDS have different components which include noninvasive evaluation (uroflowmetry) and invasive evaluation (filling cystometry, pressure–flow studies and/or urethral function measurements.) UDS may be complemented by simultaneous electromyography recording and/or X-rays (video-urodynamic study).

The classic concept of non-invasive urodynamics is related to the study of urine flow (uroflowmetry,) as the first approach. The importance of urinary flow and bladder conditions have been studied for a long time. Brodie in 1849 suggested that enlargement of the prostate contributed to weakness of the stream in older men, but postulated stricture disease was the primary factor. Young and Davis in 1926 reviewed 1000 patients with BPH and found 86 % had a weak urinary stream, but they had no devices to quantitate the strength of the stream beyond the simple clinical observation that "much can often be learned by watching the act of micturition. The size, force, character, and curve of the urinary stream often indicate the amount of obstruction that is present". Independently, Havelock Ellis In 1902, Schwartz in 1922, and Ballenger in 1932 reported the clinical importance of the cast distance of the stream. Ballenger recommended measurement of the distance of stream

---

O.A. Storme, M.D. • K.A. McCammon, M.D. (✉)
Department of Urology, Eastern Virginia Medical School, 225 Clearfield Ave.,
Virginia Beach, VA 23462, USA
e-mail: ostormec@gmail.com; mccammka@evms.edu

projection for men to monitor individual voiding capabilities and suggested urological treatment when the voiding distance decreased to less than half of previously measured individual specific values. Sigematu described a slit-flow clock device to measure urine flow and hypothesized that the device would not have much diagnostic value but might be of use prognostically. In 1948 Drake constructed the first practical uroflowmeter (UFM)using a toy erector set and a screen door spring. The device plotted accumulated urinary weight during voiding against time to produce a flow curve from which a peak flow rate could be calculated. It was improved later by Kaufman (1957). Van Garrelts constructed the first UFM that plotted a flow rate derived electrically from the flow curve. Many other ingenious methods of flow assessment ensued; among these were utilization of an electromagnetic field (Cardus in 1963), air displacement (Holm in 1962), rotating trays, acoustic techniques, and droplet dispersal analysis. Other simple but ineffective systems have also been described [2–4]. As interpretation of the data was needed, the nomograms of Siroky offered valuable information of normal and abnormal flow rates.

While invasive pressure-flow studies are the gold standard for the study ofbladder function and dysfunction,in the last years investigators have studied alternative non-invasive ways to measure bladder behavior. These will be discussed although they are not yet validated as replacements.

Uroflowmetry

Uroflowmetry is a non-invasive study, in which the patient voids into a flowmeter asurine flow rate iscontinuously measured as volume per time (ml/s) and flow is plotted with volume on the X axis and time corresponds to the Y axis [1–5].

It is possibly the most frequently used UDS because it is non-invasive and is usually the first study to evaluate voiding function; thus it is a very important instrument in the urology office [6]. The UFM does not reproduce symptoms as the UDS does, it simply measures flow. Significantly, the unnatural office environment is an awkward place for patients to recreate their normal pattern of micturition. In order to produce accurate results of testing, an effort to create a calm and relaxed atmosphere is paramount to reduce artifact in testing (Fig. 1).

Indications

Prior to invasive UDS, it is important to do non-invasive UFM. Without a catheter, evaluation of flow is more accurate than during the pressure-flow study [7]. Indications for UFM include initial evaluation of patients with benign prostatic hypertrophy, urinary incontinence, urethral strictures, recurrent urinary tract infections and neurogenic bladder dysfunction. In patients with LUTS, UFM may suggest an abnormality of voiding/emptying [8]. UFM has also been very helpful in follow up of patient status post urethroplasty in determining stricture recurrence.

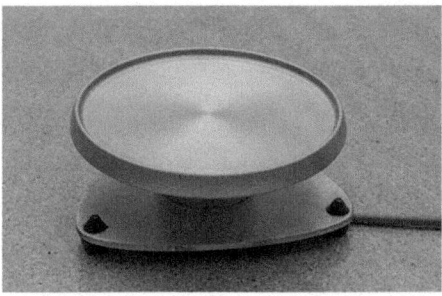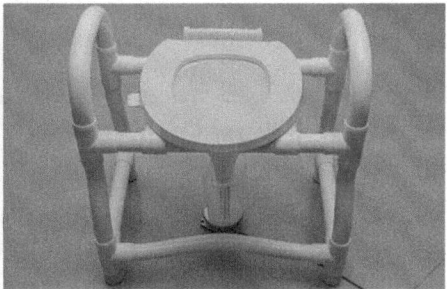

Fig. 1 Uroflowmeter (*right*), complete voiding equipment with funnel and chair (*left*). During uroflowmetry patient must void as usually does

Equipment

Types of Uroflowmeters

1. Weight: A load cell transducer measures voided weight and differentiates it with respect to time to determine the flow rate.
2. Electrical capacitance: A dipstick mounted in a collecting chamber measures the electrical capacitance. The output of the signal is proportional to the accumulated volume, and the volumetric flow rate is determined by differentiation.
3. Rotating disc: The urine stream is directed onto a rotating disc which has the power necessary to keep it rotating at a constant rate is measured with the power (in unit of measure) proportional to the flow rate (in ml/s).

Preparation

The preparation of the patient and the room are very important to reproduce a normal void. The patient should know he/she will void into an uroflowmeter (per their usual habit) usually standing up or sitting down. The patient should also be made aware of the importance of the exam to evaluate voiding symptoms. Ideally, the exam would be done with normal desire to void (preferably first desire to void), not under urgency. Bladder overdistention could alter normal flow and increase post void residual (PVR.) Theoretically you need three UFM measurements to confirm a reliable result.

The UDS room must be comfortable and silent. Unintended inability to void or artifacts can occur because of an unfamiliar environment. Sometimes it helps to leave the patient alone, turn off the lights and turn on the water.

Uroflowmetry Technique

Paper speed of 0.25 cm/s is the standard, as it allows an accurate and systematic curve construction. Different paper speeds change curve shapes, and thus can alter the interpretation of the test. Urinary flow and PRV depends on bladder urinary volume. **For accuracy of testing, voided volume must be over 150 ml and ideally less than 400–500 cc as the detrusor muscle may become overstretched and contractility may decrease, consequently creating a false result.**

Uroflowmetry Interpretation

A UFM report must include the curve description, voided volume, maximum flow rate (Q Max), average flow rate (Q Ave) and postvoid residual (PVR) to be complete.

Standard Terminology Related to UFM [9]

1. Urine Flow is described either as continuous, intermittent or fluctuant. **The continuous flow curve is represented as a smooth arc shaped curve without interruptions.** Intermittent flow is when the flow stops and starts in a repeated pattern. The curve is fluctuating when there are multiple peaks during a period of continuous urine flow without dropping off completely as in the intermittent curve pattern. **While the precise shape of the flow curve may be affected by detrusor contractility, possible bladder outlet obstruction, urethral obstruction, and or the presence of any abdominal straining, one cannot make these diagnoses without the pressure flow study on the shape of the curve alone.**
2. Flow rate is defined as the volume of fluid expelled via the urethra per unit time expressed in ml/s.
3. Voided volume is the total volume expelled via the urethra.
4. Maximum flow rate is the maximum measured value of the flow rate after correction for artifacts (ml/s).
5. Voiding time is the total duration of micturition, including interruptions. When a void is completed without interruption, voiding time is equal to flow time.
6. Flow time is the time over which measurable flow actually occurs. Men average approximately 30 s and women average approximately 20 s to void.
7. Average flow rate is volume divided by flow time. The average flow should be interpreted with caution if flow is interrupted or if there is a terminal dribble.
8. Time to maximum flow is the elapsed time from onset of flow to maximum flow.
9. Post void residual (PVR) is defined as the volume of urine left in the bladder at the end of micturition determined by either ultrasound or catheterization. If there is no demonstrated PVR after repeated free flowmetry, then the finding of residual urine during the UDS should be considered an artifact.

10. Bladder outletobstruction is the general term for obstruction during micturition characterized by increased detrusor pressure and reduced urine flow rate. It is usually diagnosed by studying the synchronous values of flow rate and detrusor pressure. BOO has been defined for men, but as yet, not adequately quantified in women and children (see chapter "The Pressure Flow Study" for more information).
11. Dysfunctional voiding is an intermittent and/or fluctuating flow rate due to involuntary intermittent contractions of the periurethral striated muscle during micturition in neurologically normal individuals.

Normal Values

In adult males Q max ≤ 10 ml/s, UFM has a specificity of 70–90 %, with a PPV of 70 % and a sensitivity of 39–47 % to diagnosis obstruction [10, 11].

Common causes of BOO in woman include pelvic organ prolapse, iatrogenic obstruction after incontinence surgery and pelvic masses [12]. Women BOO values are not standardized. UFM excludes BOO in women with Q max > 15 ml/s, voided volume > 100 ml, normal curve and no significant postvoid residual [13], but pressure-flow nomogram defined obstruction if Q max < 12 ml/s and Pdet Q max > 20 cm H_2O [14].

Curves

Urine flow results from a detrusor contraction and urethral resistance, thus changes in flow curves imply an imbalance between these factors. While a noninvasive flow test is a good screening test for voiding dysfunction, one must remember the only way to definitively diagnose these issues is through pressure flow studies (see chapter "The Pressure Flow Study").

1. Normal Curve: Is continuous and has a bell shape, Q max is reached in the first third of the tracing and within 3–10 s from the start of flow. The final phase shows a rapid fall from high flow together with a sharp cutoff at the end of flow (Fig. 2).
2. Continuous Flow Curves (Fig. 3):
   – Bladder outlet obstruction: This type of curve has an elongated shape in benign prostatic obstruction (compressive). It appears normal in the first third but has a reduced Qmax with the latter part of the curve elongated with a terminal dribble indicating a reduction in flow rate. In the presence of urethral stricture (constrictive), the curve is plateau-shaped with little, change between Qmax and Qave.
   – With idiopathic detrusor overactivity a supranormal curve for high detrusor contraction velocities is observed. The curve is of normal shape with a very high Q max, within 1–3 s of the initial flow.
   – With detrusor underactivity the diagnosis is cystometric. UFM shows a symmetrical tracing with low Q max. The time to reach Q max is variable, and Q

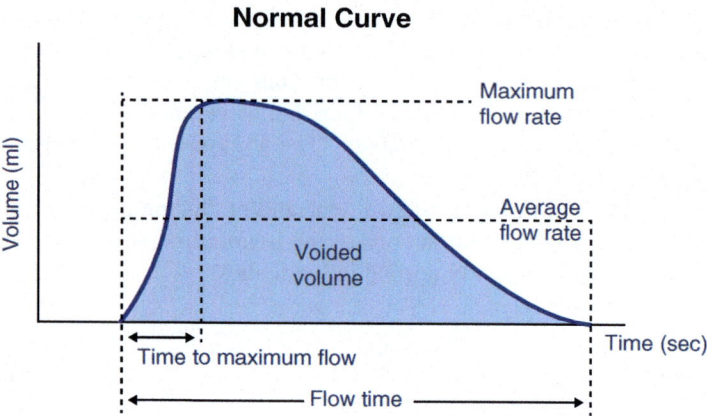

Fig. 2 Illustration of normal curve, continuous and bell shape, Q max is reached in the first third and final phase shows a rapid fall from high flow together with a sharp cutoff at the end

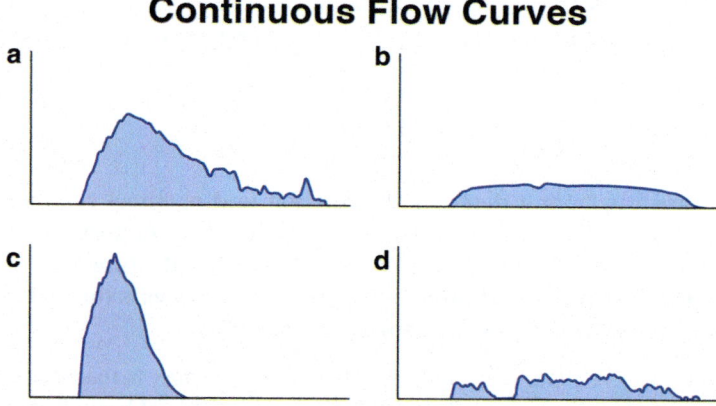

Fig. 3 (**a**) Compressive flow curve (benign prostatic obstruction); (**b**) Constrictive flow curve (urethral stricture); (**c**) Idiopathic detrusor overactivity; (**d**) Detrusor underactivity

max may occur in the second half of the curve. If these features appear in UFM, a pressure-flow study must be done.

3. Intermittent flow curve (Fig. 4):

   - Normal patients: Sawtooth curve, similar to DSD in neurologically normal patient, most often a result of anxiety or dysfunctional voiding.
   - Detrusor sphincter dyssynergia: Sawtooth curve in neurologically abnormal patient with involuntary external sphincter contraction alongside bladder contraction.

Intermittent Flow Curves

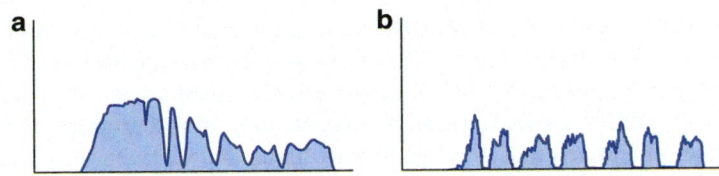

Fig. 4 (a) Detrusor sphincter dyssynergia; (b) Valsalva voiding curve: patients with areflexic or hypocontractile bladder void with valsalva maneuver that is represented as an intermittent and irregular curve

- Areflexic bladder: Patients can void with (crede) valsava maneuver, in other cases the contraction is poorly sustained or fluctuates as in multiple sclerosis.

Complementary Study to UFM

Post Void Residual (PVR)

The post-void residual (PVR) may be measured noninvasively by ultrasound or invasively by catheterization. It is often used as a complement to UFM in patients with LUTS, initially and during follow up. **An elevated PVR may indicate detrusor underactivity, BOO or both. There is no agreement upon a standard definition of exactly what volume constitutes an elevated PVR, therefore this alone cannot be used to differentiate between an obstructed or unobstructed patient** [8–15].

New Alternatives to Non-invasive Methods

Investigators have tried to find noninvasive techniques to assess voiding pressure by measuring isovolumetric bladder pressure without a catheter therefore allowing the patient to void without the possible obstruction by the UDS catheter. **While the gold standard remains the pressure-flow study, this may be expensive, uncomfortable for the patient and has approximately 5 % risk of symptomatic urine infection** [16].

Bladder/Detrusor Wall Thickness (DWT)

DWT has been studied as a non-invasive approach to BOO, because it is associated with detrusor hypertrophy leading to increased wall thickness. However, the bladder thickness can be overestimated for mucosal diseases such as tumors or infection. Hence, DWT could be an accurate alternative, but may be inappropriate in the presence of other conditions that increase fibrous tissue and collagen that occur naturally with age versus obstruction [15–17]. Animal studies confirm that detrusor hypertrophy decreases after relief of obstruction. In normal patients, DWT decreases quickly initially and then stabilizes [18]. DWT could detect BOO in a noninvasive way and may predict the potential responsiveness to alpha blocker treatment for LUTS in men [19], but the cutoff measurement is not well defined. Some studies propose DTW of 2 mm or over, yet other studies show no differences between obstructed and non-obstructed patients [20–23].

Penile Cuff Test

In this test, the cuff is placed around the penis and is inflated and deflated while the patient voids into a urine flowmeter. Two methods have been studied. McRae et al. modeled their test on conventional blood pressure measurement. The urethra was occluded with a small inflatable cuff applying uniform circumferential pressure. He proposes a simple noninvasive technique that measures maximum (isovolumetric) bladder pressure in the absence of flow, then measures the maximum flow rate under optimum conditions. The patient is then instructed to void. The urethra becomes distended with urine proximal to the occluding cuff such that the static proximal intraurethral pressure is related proportionally to the maximum (isovolumetric) bladder pressure. The recorded isovolumetric pressure, the urinary flow rate and the flow rate waveform provide information that theoretically relates to detrusor performance, the carrying capacity of the urethra, and the location of urinary blockage. However, only a single measurement is obtained and false readings can occur [24].

Griffiths et al. developed another technique that utilizes controlled inflation of a penile cuff. Known as the interruption technique, after micturition begins the cuff is inflated until flow is interrupted. The cuff pressure is measured at this point and then is rapidly deflated to allow micturition to resume. This cycle can be repeated until voiding ends. The new noninvasive measurement is compared with bladder pressure measured in a simultaneous invasive pressure flow study. In healthy volunteers and patients the mean cuff pressure overestimated the bladder pressure by 14.5 ± 14 cm H_2O. A nomogram was constructed to classify obstructed and non-obstructed patients [25]. Inter-observer studies conclude that there is reasonable agreement between experienced observers in their interpretation of data from the cuff test [26], but in the SIU international consultation of LUTS in men, there is no recommendation yet possible [8].

Condom Catheter Method (CCM)

In this method the patient voids through an incontinence condom fitted with a pressure catheter. The patient voids into the closed catheter and at maximum flow the catheter is blocked and isovolumetric pressure is measured [27]. Infravesical obstruction can be diagnosed using the pressure recorded by the condom catheter and the Qmax from a separately measured free flow rate utilizing a classification strategy which has been previously validated [8]. CCM reproducibility is comparable to that of conventional invasive methods, with a success rate of 94 % and a reproducibility comparable to that of invasive pressure flow studies [28]. A similar device has been studied with the sensitivity and specificity for BOO of 67 % and 79 %, respectively [29]. In comparative PFS the accuracy of agreement is only 65 % for the ICS obstructed group alone, a value that should be compared with accuracies of 82–83 % for PFS's themselves [8–30]. With regard to SIU international consultation of LUTS in men there is no recommendation on this method yet possible [8].

Near Infrared Spectroscopy (NIRS)

Near infrared spectroscopy (NIRS) measures changes in bladder blood flow (chromofore concentration using infrared light) during micturion. NIRS measures oxyhemoglobin and deoxyhemoglobin levels in tissues. The theory is that during micturition in normal or unobstructed patients a reactive hyperemia occurs. In obstructed bladders, the detrusor muscle increases oxygen consumption, the oxyhemoglobin and deoxyhemoglobin levels are lower and there is less hyperemia. However, actual studies have demonstrated contradictory results. Some studies promised sensitivity and specificity to predict BOO of over 80 % of the time in men with LUTS. Although other studies show that the near infrared spectroscopy pattern component itself did not correlate strongly with obstruction [31]. Thus, more investigation is necessary for standardization and technology application for further use of this method [8–17].

Conclusions

Uroflowmetry is a noninvasive urodynamic study and should be one of the initial approaches to clinically evaluate voiding symptoms. The parameters of volume of urine voided, shape of the flow curve and the maximum flow rate are very important for the understanding of the etiology of a patients LUTS, but pressure-flow study remains the gold standard for BOO diagnosis. New NIU studies are promising as alternatives, but are not yet validated for general use.

References

1. Abrams P. Urodynamics. 3rd ed. London: Springer; 2006. p. 17–39.
2. Bowley A, Legg W. A new uroflowmeter-an instrument for the estimation of liquid volume and rate of flow. Med Biol Eng. 1971;9(2):139–42.
3. Chancellor M, Rivas D, Mulholland S, Drake W. The invention of the modern uroflowmeter by Willard M. Drake Jr. At Jefferson Medical College. Urology. 1998;51(4):671–4.
4. Bloom D, Foster W, McLeod D, Mittmeyer B, Stutzman R. Cost-effective uroflowmetry in men. J Urol. 1985;133(3):421–4.
5. Abrams P, Cardozo L, Khoury S, Wein A. Incontinence. 4th International Consultation on Incontinence, Paris, 5–8 July; 2008. p. 418–9.
6. Shäfer W, Abrams P, Liao L, Mattiasson A, Pesce F, Spangberg A, Sterling A, Zinner N, Van Kerrebroeck P. Good urodynamic practices: uroflowmetry, filling cystometry, and pressure-flow studies. Neurourol Urodyn. 2002;21:261–74.
7. Richard P, Icaza N, Mai TL. The effect of a 6 french catheter on flow rate in men. Urol Ann. 2013;5(4):264–8.
8. Chapple C, Abrams P. International consultation on male LUTS, SIU. 2012. Comitee 2. p. 37–133.
9. Abrams P, Cardozo L, Fall M, Griffiths D, Rosier P, Ulmsten U, Van Kerrebroeck P, Victor A, Wein A. The standardisation of terminology of lower urinary tract function: report from the standardisation sub-committee of the International Continence Society. Neurourol Urodyn. 2002;21:167–78.
10. Reynard J, Yang Q, Donovan J, Peters T, Schafer W, De la Rosette J, Dabhoiwala N, Osawa D, Tong Long Lim A, Abrams P. The ICS "BPH" Study: uroflowmetry, lower urinary tract symptoms and bladder outlet obstruction. Br J Urol. 1998;82(5):619–23.
11. Reynard J, Peters T, Lim C, Abrams P. The value of multiple free-flow studies in men with lower urinary tract symptoms. Br J Urol. 1996;77:813–8.
12. Nitti V. Pressure flow urodynamic studies: the gold standard for diagnosing bladder outlet obstruction. Rev Urol. 2005;7 Suppl 6:S14–21.
13. Bass J, Leach G. Bladder outlet obstruction in women. Prob Urol. 1991;5:141–54.
14. Blaivas J, Groutz A. Bladder outlet obstruction nomogram for women with lower urinary tract symptomatology. Neurourol Urodyn. 2000;19:553–64.
15. Winter J, Dmochowski R, Goldman H, et al. Urodynamic studies in adult: AUA/SUFU guideline. J Urol. 2012;188(6 Suppl):2464–72.
16. Klinger H, Madersbacher S, Djavan B, et al. Morbidity of the evaluation of the lower urinary tract with transurethral multichannel pressure-flow studies. J Urol. 1998;159:191.
17. Sahai A, Seth J, Van der Aa F, Panicker J, De Ridder D, Dasgupta P. Current state of the art in non-invasive urodynamics. Curr Bladder Dysfunct Rep. 2013;8:83–91.
18. Saito M, Ohmura M, Kondo A. Effects of long-term partial outflow obstruction on bladder function in the rat. Neurourol Urodyn. 1996;15(2):157–65.
19. Park J, Lee H, Lee S, Moon H, Park H, Kim Y. Bladder wall thickness is associated with responsiveness of storage symptoms to alpha-blockers in men with lower urinary tract symptoms. Kor J Urol. 2012;53:487–91.
20. Oelke M, Höfner K, Jonas U, De la Rosette J, Ubbink D, Wijkstra H. Diagnostic accuracy of noninvasive test to evaluate bladder outlet obstruction in men: detrusor wall thickness, uroflowmetry, postvoid residual urine, and prostate volume. Eur Urol. 2007;52:827–35.
21. Kessler T, Gerber R, Burkhard F, Studer U, Danuser H. Ultrasound assessment of detrusor thickness in men—can it predict bladder outlet obstruction and replace pressure flow study? J Urol. 2006;175(6):2170–3.
22. Belal M, Abrams P. Noninvasive methods of diagnosing bladder outlet obstruction in men. Part 1: Nonurodynamic approach. J Urol. 2006;176:22.
23. Oelke M. International Consultation on Incontinence-Research Society (ICI-RS) report on non-invasive urodynamics: the need of standardization of ultrasound bladder and detrusor wall

thickness measurements to quantify bladder wall hypertrophy. Neurourol Urodyn. 2010; 29:634–9.
24. McRae L, Bottaccini M, Gleason D. Noninvasive quantitative method for measuring isovolumetric bladder pressure and urethral resistance in the male: experimental validation of the theory. Neurourol Urodyn. 1995;14:101.
25. Griffiths C, et al. Noninvasive measurement of bladder pressure by controlled inflation of a penile cuff. J Urol. 2002;167(3):1344–7.
26. Drinnan M, McIntosh S, Robson W, Pickard R, Ramsden P, Clive J. Inter-observer agreement in the estimation of bladder pressure using a penile cuff. Neurourol Urodyn. 2003;22:296–300.
27. Gommer E, Vanspauwen T, Miklosi M, Wen J, Kinder M, Janknegt R, Van Waalwijk van Doorn E. Validity of a non-invasive determination of the isovolumetric bladder pressure during voiding in men with LUTS. Neurourol Urodyn. 1999;18:477–86.
28. Huang Foen Chung J, Bohnen A, Pel J, Bosch J, Niesing R, Van Mastrigt R. Applicability and reproducibility of condom catheter method for measuring isovolumetric bladder pressure. Urology. 2004;63:56–60.
29. Levi C, Magalhães J, De Oliveira F, Carvalho J, Oliveira R, Netto N. New method for minimally invasive urodynamic assessment in men with lower urinary tract symptoms. Urology. 2008;71:75–8.
30. Pel J, Bosch J, Blom J, Lycklama à Nijeholt A, Van Mastrigt R. Development of a non-invasive strategy to classify bladder outlet obstruction in male patients with LUTS. Neurourol Urodyn. 2002;21(2):117–25.
31. Chung D, Lee R, Kaplan S, Te A. Concordance of near infrared spectroscopy with pressure flow studies in men with lower urinary tract symptoms. J Urol. 2010;184(6):2434–9.

The Cystometrogram

Ryan L. Steinberg and Karl J. Kreder

Introduction

The cystometrogram is the most comprehensive means of assessing the bladder's ability to store urine and activity during filling. Bladder and rectal pressures during testing should be performed with a transurethral catheter and a separate rectal balloon catheter with external pressure transducer, per International Continence Society guidelines. The detrusor pressure can then be calculated by subtracting the abdominal pressure from the intravesical pressure. Saline, water, or cystografin (when performing videourodynamics) should be used to fill the bladder at a rate of 0–100 mL/min. The cystometrogram is closely monitored in real time during filling to assess for decreased bladder compliance, which if left addressed, can lead to upper urinary tract deterioration over time. Provocative maneuvers, including a cough, Valsalva maneuver, and running water, may be employed to elicit detrusor overactivity. The administration of provocative medications during filling, such as bethanechol, is no long employed and are now only of historical interest. Leak point pressures can also be determined to evaluate for stress urinary incontinence and neurogenic bladders. Abnormally elevated pressures encountered during cystometry usually arise from the rectal catheter and may be related to catheter positioning.

R.L. Steinberg, M.D. (✉) • K.J. Kreder, M.D.
Department of Urology, University of Iowa,
200 Hawkins Dr., 3 RCP, Iowa City, IA 52242-1089, USA
e-mail: RyanSteinbergMD@gmail.com; karl-kreder@uiowa.edu

Procedural Preparation

Bladder Catheter

Bladder Catheter After the patient has completed noninvasive flow studies, he/she is asked to lie supine on the fluoroscopy table. If the patient was unable to void during the prior study or has a history of significant urinary retention (>200 mL), a straight catheter, typically a 14 Fr red rubber, is inserted in standard sterile fashion to maximally drain the bladder. If the patient was able to void and does not have a significant history of urinary retention, the test catheter can simply be placed without need for straight catheterization.

There are numerous commercially available catheters that exist for urodynamic testing. The major distinction to make amongst these catheters is the means of pressure measurement. The external pressure transducer with fluid-filled catheter was first described by Brown and Wicksham in 1969 and was the standard by which urodynamic techniques were developed [1]. This device functions by sensing changes in the vesical pressure which can be transmitted via non-compressible sterile water or saline within the catheter channel and applied to an external strain gauge. **An essential element to using these types of catheters, or any external transduction equipment, is to ensure that the transducer is mounted at the superior edge of the pubic symphysis perInternational Continence Society (ICS)guidelines** [2]. Failure to place the transducer at the same level as the bladder will result in erroneously high (if below the level of the bladder) or low (if above the level of the bladder) pressures. Advantages of these catheters are that they are low cost and disposable, thus negating the need to sterilize the equipment and minimizing lost testing time. Disadvantages include the potential for signal artifact with patient movement, kinks in the catheter, and obstruction from intraluminal air within the catheter.

Another option for pressure measurement is to utilize an air-charged catheter with an external pressure transducer. This functions in a similar manner as the water-filled catheter except with a small balloon overlying the catheter tip to ensure separation from the bladder wall. The catheter is filled with air and thus, pressure is transmitted directly from the catheter tip to the transducer. Placement of the external transducer at the level of the bladder remains critical to accurate measurements. Advantages of these catheters are that there is very little motion artifact created by movement of the line, making this advantageous during studies including walking or movements. Disadvantages include a slowed response and attenuation of the transmitted signal to the transducer, thus leading to an overdampened system [3].

The final means of pressure measurement is a catheter-tip transducer (Micro-Tip Catheter). This was first described by Millar and Baker in 1973 for measurement of aortic-pressure pulse waves [4]. It was later introduced into urodynamics for vesical and urethral pressure measurements by Asmussen and Ulmsten in 1975 [5]. Pressures are measured by a transducer mounted on the tip of the catheter, which detect changes by means of strain. This is converted into an electric signal (voltage), which can later be amplified and transmitted to a semiconductor for conversion into a pressure measurement (the voltage and pressure measurements are proportional to one another). One advantage of this method of pressure measurement is a faster equipment response in detecting pressure changes, leading to more accurate real-time measurements and a reliable means of evaluating the Valsalva leak point pressure [5]. Furthermore, minimal motion artifact makes these catheters superior to water-filled catheters when conducting ambulatory urodynamics [6]. Unfortunately, the significant expense of these catheters, given the miniature nature of the transducers, the need for sterilization/reuse of these catheters, cost, and the inability to confirm consistent positioning during the entire study are major disadvantages. The latter is important to consider as significant intravesical pressure variability can occur (up to 10 cm H_2O difference between the dome and base). **The ICS recommends a fluid-filled catheter with external transducer for routine urodynamic testing** [7].

Each of these catheters can be purchased in a wide variety of sizes (6–10 Fr), number of lumens (1–3), and tips (straight, Tiemann, pigtail). Catheter size should be minimized to prevent the possibility of outflow obstruction from the catheter during the voiding phase of the study. Studies evaluating the level of obstruction from various sized catheters used during urodynamics, which is of particular importance with obstructive conditions such as BPH, have all demonstrated reduced flow rates, but actual results regarding true obstruction have been varied [8–10]. **There has also been the practice of placing two, single lumen catheters, one large bore catheter for filling and a second small caliber catheter for pressure transduction. The reasoning behind this method is to allow for higher filling rates given the larger diameter catheter, which can later be removed, and minimize any obstructive effects by using a small caliber pressure catheter.** Unfortunately, removal of the larger catheter does not allow for repeat filling/testing to be accomplished without replacement of the catheter which is both invasive and uncomfortable.

Walker et al. evaluated suprapubic pressure measurements to examine the possibility of obstruction from a transurethral catheter [11]. While this study did demonstrate a statistically significant difference in the maximum flow rate and detrusor pressure at maximum flow rate and thus changes to the severity grading of obstruction, the clinical significance of these numerical differences are negligible and changes in obstruction grading appear to be arbitrary. Suprapubic measurements may still prove to be the optimal means of assessing bladder function in patients with urethral stricture disease and selected infants, though in practice this is quite rare. The number of lumens is dictated by the number of parameters attempting to be recorded. A catheter with the least number of lumens as needed should be used to minimize the pressure signal dampening which can occur with small caliber lumen. Also, filling rate limitations can be encountered with smaller catheters. Depending on the means by which the inflow volume is recorded, erroneous measurements of the volume instilled can be recorded. **The ICS recommends a transurethral double-lumen catheter to be used for routine urodynamics** [7]. Our institution routinely utilizes a 6 Fr transurethral double-lumen fluid-filled catheter with external transducer (Fig. 1).

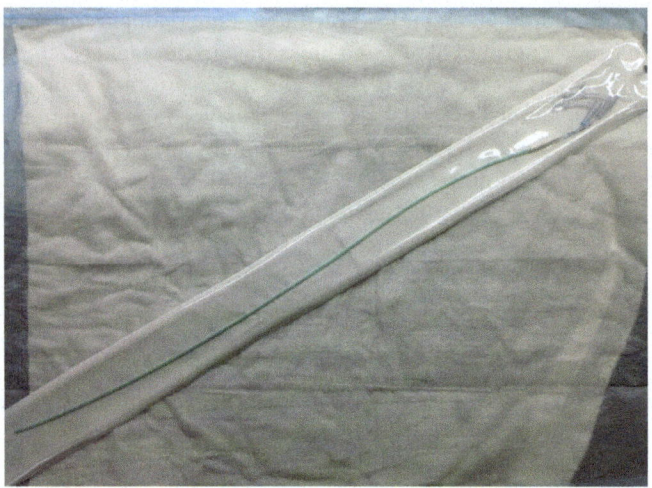

Fig. 1 A 6 Fr dual lumen urethral catheter for urodynamic testing

Bladder Catheter Placement

After the above mentioned catheter is obtained, the patient is prepped and draped in normal sterile fashion and the catheter is inserted. Typically, plain water-based lubrication can be utilized for insertion. In certain circumstances, such as patients with urethral/pelvic pain, significant anxiety, or a history of difficult catheterization, 5–10 mL of 2 % lidocaine jelly may be injected into the urethra and allowed to anesthetize the urethra for up to 5 min prior to catheter insertion. After placement, any residual urine within the bladder is then allowed to drain until the bladder is empty. The catheter is then secured by paper tape placed on the dorsal aspect of the penis and wrapped around the catheter in men and on the medial thigh in women. In patients with catheterizable channels, the transurethral catheter is placed through the channel and taped to the abdominal wall. The pressure transducer is then taped to the patient's side at the level of the superior edge of the pubic symphysis, even with the height of the bladder. The atmospheric cap on the opposite end of the transducer is removed then opening the transducer to the atmosphere. Using a three-way stopcock, the transducer is flushed and zeroed using the computer software (Fig. 2). The atmospheric cap is then replaced. The stopcock is then rotated and the connection tubing between the transducer and catheter is flushed to remove any air bubbles. The tubing is then connected to the catheter. The baseline intravesical pressure is assessed to confirm appropriate placement (typically 0–5 cm H_2O). A cough is used to confirm good signal transmission.

Regardless of the type of catheter placed, zeroing of the urethral catheter to the atmosphere prior to initiation of any study with any type of catheter is

The Cystometrogram

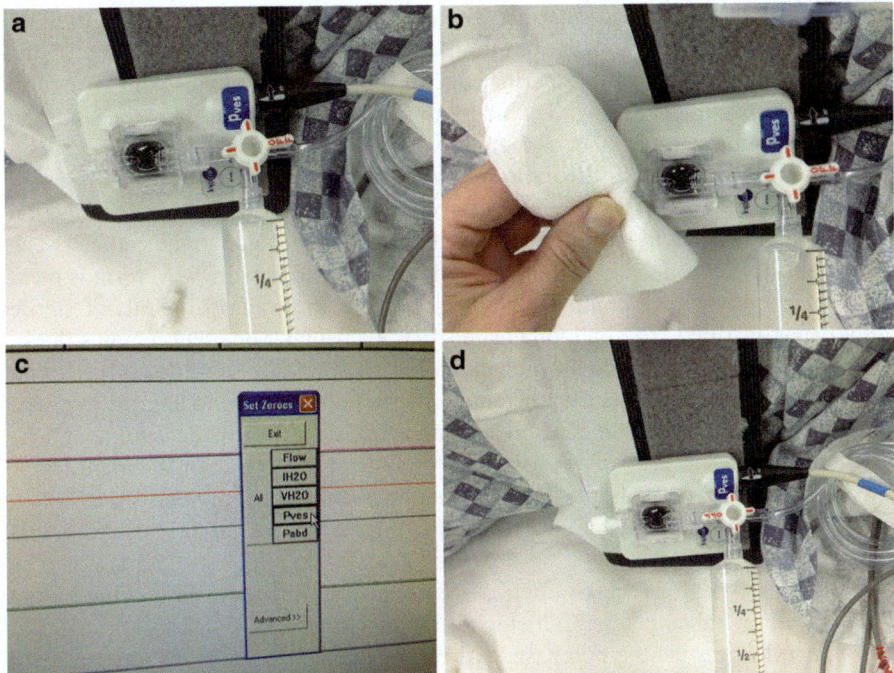

Fig. 2 (**a**) Three-way stopcock set up for zeroing the transducer (atmospheric cap already removed). (**b**) Flushing the transducer with saline. (**c**) Zeroing the flushed transducer which is open to the atmosphere. (**d**) Capping the transducer and flushing the connection tubing to the catheter

paramount and strongly recommended in the ICS guidelines. More recently, there has been increasing difficulty in identifying the upper border of the pubic symphysis with the ongoing obesity epidemic occurring worldwide. In light of this, many urodynamics labs have begun to zero the pressure transducer once within the patient's bladder. This is strongly opposed by the ICS. This does not allow for a resting intravesical and abdominal pressure to be obtained, which can be variable in patients. Further, intracorporal zeroing may cause the abdominal pressure to become zero during the voiding phase as the pelvic floor relaxes, which can skew the results of the detrusor pressure [7].

Rectal Catheter Placement

After placement of the urethral catheter, the rectal catheter can then be placed. The catheter is well lubricated, inserted into the anus, and advanced ~4 cm. The abdominal pressure transducer is part of a multi-transducer apparatus, along with the intravesical transducer, and thus has already been placed at the time of urethral catheter placement. As with the urethral catheter, appropriate positioning of the transducer at the level of the superior edge of the pubic symphysis is important to obtaining an accurate reading. The abdominal pressure transducer is then flushed and zeroed in the same manner as the intravesical pressure transducer. **As has been previously stated, zeroing the catheter to the atmosphere and not the intracorporeal baseline pressure is critical to accurate measurements.** The connection tubing is then flushed to remove any air bubbles and connected to the catheter. The balloon of the rectal catheter is then inflated until a good pressure waveform is present on the urodynamics computer software, with a maximum of 2 mL of sterile saline being instilled. The balloon ensures that the catheter opening remains unobstructed by surrounding feces, which can affect the pressure sensation. Overfilling of the balloon can lead to elastic distention of the balloon surrounding the pressure transducer and thus result in a falsely elevated baseline pressure measurement. The baseline intravesical pressure is assessed to confirm appropriate placement (typically 0–5 cm H_2O). A cough or Valsalva can be used to confirm good signal transmission. The catheter is secured in placed using paper tape on the posteromedial aspect of the right thigh.

Numerous types of rectal catheters are commercially available, similar to the options for ureteral catheters. Catheters of various lumens (1–3), sizes (from 4.5 to 21 Fr), and lengths can be purchased. At our institution, we manufacture our own rectal catheters for urodynamic testing (Fig. 3). These are produced by first cutting the fingers off of a silicone glove. These silicone pieces are placed over the cut end of 14 Fr IV tubing to act as a balloon. A 12 Fr Foley catheter is then cut into cross-sectional rings, and using a hemostat, these rings are placed over the balloon and advanced 2–3 cm from the cut end of the IV tubing. This provides a watertight seal to the balloon. This catheter is attached to a three-way stopcock which can be connected to the pressure transducer. These institution-produced rectal catheters have proven to be effective both with regards to pressure measurements and cost (estimated cost of each assembled catheter is $1).

Using rectal pressure measurements to estimate intraabdominal pressure has long been considered the gold standard [12]. The rectum is an optimal point of measurement given its low baseline pressures (4 cm H_2O) and good wall compliance, thus minimizing any rectal generated pressures from being transmitted [13]. More recently, intra-vaginal pressure measurements have also been investigated as an alternative given the greater comfort of a vaginal catheter in women. Results have been largely supportive of accurate pressure transmission [14, 15] with the exception of one study which found a statistically significant difference in the vaginal and rectal pressures in specific situations (changes in positioning and filling) [16]. While significant, the mean pressure difference was only 3.0–3.33 cm H_2O, and thus the clinical applicability of an intra-vaginal means of pressure measurement seems reasonable. **The International Continence Society continues to recommend a rectal balloon catheter in the measurement of the abdominal pressure.**

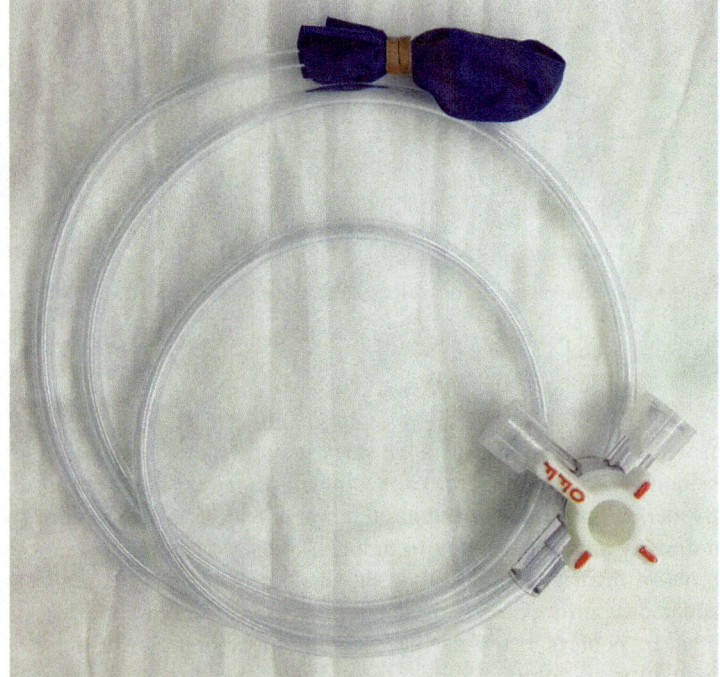

Fig. 3 A simply constructed rectal catheter for urodynamic testing

Determining Detrusor Pressure

The detrusor pressure (Pdet) is a calculated value based upon the pressures sensed from the intravesical (Pves) and rectal (Pabd) catheters. The concept of detrusor pressure stems from the fact that the intravesical pressure is a combination of the pressure generated by the detrusor muscle of the bladder/bladder wall, as well as transmitted abdominal pressure created by abdominal musculature. Pressure generated by the detrusor muscle or bladder wall can be isolated by subtracting the abdominal pressure as measured in a different location, in this case the rectum: **Pdet = Pves − Pabd.**

The Cystometrogram

Filling

Once both catheters have been placed and good signal transmission is appreciated, bladder filling can commence. Normally, the fluoroscopy table is gradually tilted to 90° (patient upright) during the initial filling (Fig. 4). However, in certain cases such

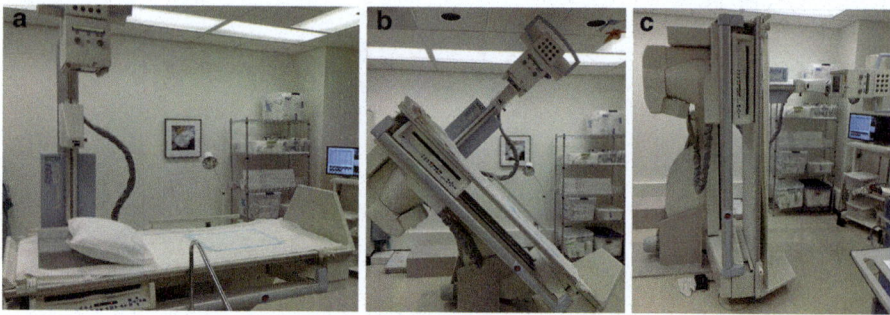

Fig. 4 Sequential patient positioning during filling from supine (**a**), to 45° (**b**), to upright (**c**)

as patients with spinal cord disorders the study may be conducted in a sitting or even supine position. There are a variety of mediums that can be used for bladder filling, including water, saline, contrast, and gas (carbon dioxide). **Saline is regarded as the closest in density and consistency to urine.** The use of carbon dioxide cystometry has fallen out of favor given that filling the bladder with air is not physiologic, can cause bladder discomfort due to dissolution of the carbon dioxide into urine and thereby create carbonic acid, and can have significant variability in testing results [17].

The instillation of contrast allows for videourodynamics to be performed and thus can simultaneously assess the bladder for structural and dynamic abnormalities during testing. However, contrast has very different chemical and physical properties compared to saline. With regard to the difference in chemical properties, cystografin is slightly acidic (pH 7.1–7.3) compared to saline [18]. Bladder reactivity to solutions of various pH values has been well documented with overactivity [19] and the desire to void at lower volumes [20] reported with acidic fluids and relaxation with larger storage capacities with alkaline solutions [21]. Cystografin is only minimally acidic compared to the solutions used in these studies and thus is felt to have no effect on bladder sensation or overactivity. Further, the density of cystografin (30 %) and cystografin dilute (18 %) compared to saline are 1.162 and 1.009 respectively, making these heavier fluids [18]. In theory, given this fact, the amount of force transmitted onto the bladder wall, and thus intravesical pressure generated, could be larger when using these agents and thus skew urodynamic results. An initial investigation revealed no differences but was methodologically flawed [22]. **A later study demonstrated that a statistically significant but minimal clinically significant elevation in the voiding detrusor pressure compared to saline** [23]. **Thus, cystografin is felt to be a viable alternative to saline for urodynamics.** The temperature of instilled fluids is also an important consideration. First described by Bors in 1957 [24] in the evaluation of neurologic insults, it has been well establish in both cats and humans that the instillation of cold fluids into the bladder incites a spinal reflex via unmyelinated C-fiber simulation and induces a detrusor contraction [25–33]. Conversely, there is minimal literature regarding instillation of warm or hot fluid into the bladder. McDonald described the primary response as pain, with a reported mean temperature of 47 °C [34]. Our institution uses room temperature cystografin for cystometry.

The next major consideration during bladder filling is the rate. Physiologic bladder filling normally occurs at a rate of 1–2 mL/min, but can increase to 10–15 mL/min with diuresis. Filling rates have been classically described as slow (less than 10 mL/min), moderate (10–100 mL/min), and fast (>100 mL/min) [35]. This nomenclature was replaced with physiologic vs. non-physiologic filling rates as per Abrams' standardization of terminology in 2002 [36]. Physiologic filling was defined as a rate less than the predicted maximum filling rate, which is derived by dividing the weight in kilograms by 4 and expressed as units of mL/min. Non-physiologic filling rates exceed this calculated value [37]. The use of body-warm saline at a physiologic filling rate is recommended in the European Association of Urology Guidelines on Neurogenic Lower Urinary Tract Dysfunction [38]. This rate is often exceeded in clinical practice. **One concern with utilizing a physiologic rate is that the actual bladder volume may be significantly different than the volume instilled due to urine production. Conversely, supraphysiologic filling rates can provoke detrusor contractions or a micturition reflex due to a rapid rise in bladder pressure. However, supraphysiologic fillingdoes not appear to affect total bladder capacity and first sensation [39, 40].** Of note, the one study that demonstrated these provoked contractions/reflexes utilized an air charged catheter and carbon dioxide for bladder filling, which as previously discussed can be very irritative to the bladder wall. This can itself induce a lower threshold for sensation and tolerability for achieve an accurate maximum capacity [41]. **Our institution routinely begins filling at 60 mL/min for adults but may reduce the rate if patients report discomfort or overactivity is felt to be induced. A reduced rate of 15–30 mL/min is utilized in patients with a history ofinterstitial cystitis/bladder pain syndrome (IC/BPS),evaluation ofoveractive bladder syndrome (OAB)and pediatric studies. A rate of 10 mL/min is used for infant evaluations.**

Provocative Measures During Filling

During filling, a number of provocative maneuvers can be performed to expose an abnormality. The most common maneuver utilized is a cough, which is used to elicit stress urinary incontinence (SUI). Diagnosis of stress urinary incontinence by means of symptomology and an office cough stress test has been shown to have poor sensitivity [42]. Formal cystometry has demonstrated both good sensitivity (81–91 %) and specificity (80–100 %) for SUI [43–45], though the evidence of an abnormal urethral pressure profile in not often present [45, 46]. Another often used maneuver is the Valsalva technique, again in an attempt to induce SUI. This will be further explored later in the leak point pressure section. Handwashing [47, 48] and heel bouncing [48, 49] has also been well documented as effective aggravating factors in the evaluation of detrusor overactivity.

Patient positioning is another important consideration, particularly in the evaluation of detrusor overactivity (DO). It is well documented that DO is more commonly elicited with standing [50–53] and sitting [49, 54], compared to a supine position. Ramsden et al. refuted these findings but did not consider rectal pressure in evaluating detrusor pressure and included pediatric patients, which likely skewed their results [55]. Other studies have found that DO can be elicited when changing positions with a full bladder or during filling bladder [56–58]. A recent review article by Al-Hayek suggested that all patients be filled sitting or standing, so as to most accurately reproduce normal filling habits and have the best opportunity to elicit detrusor overactivity [59]. Figure 5 demonstrates an example of DO elicited during testing. **Our institution utilizes cough, Valsalva, and handwashing as provocative measures. With regard to patient positioning, as filling is taking place, the fluoroscopy table is sequentially tilted until the patient is in a standing position.**

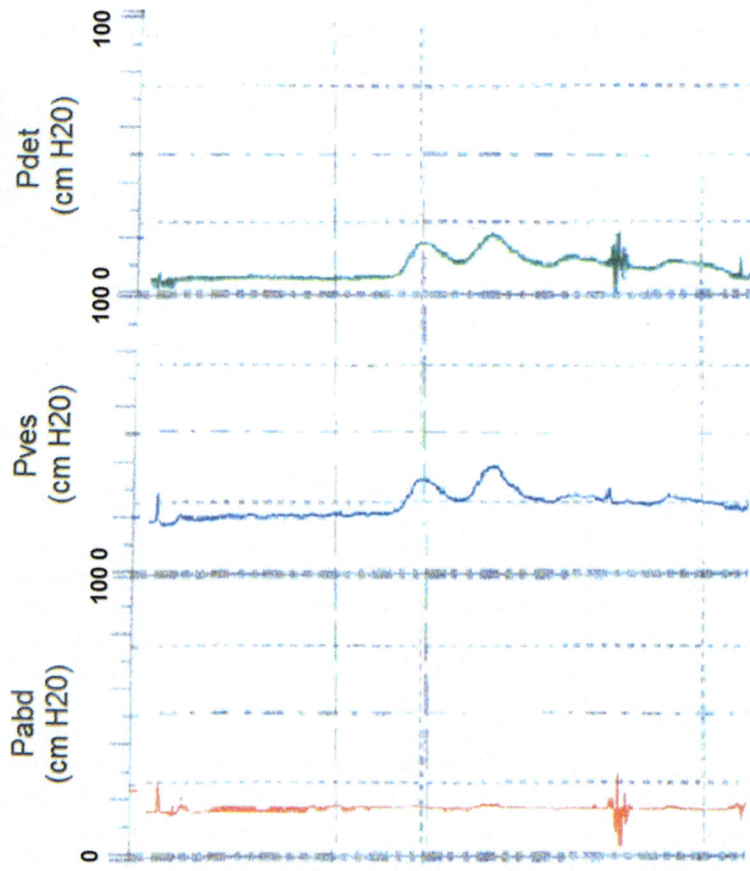

Fig. 5 Detrusor overactivity provoked during bladder filling

Sitting and walking in placearealso used in select patient populations, such as post-prostatectomy patients, to assess SUI and DO.

Administration of provocative medications have also been reported during or just prior to cystometry. Potassium chloride instillation prior to urodynamic studies has previously been reported as a means to identifying IC/BPS. This was first reported by Parsons et al. in 1998 and specifically looked to detect abnormal epithelial permeability, as is common in IC/BPS [60]. Multiple other studies confirmed that these instillations could reproduce the common symptoms of IC/BPS [61, 62], namely frequency, urgency, nocturia, and bladder pain. Unfortunately, even in the original study, 26 % of patients who met all National Institute for Diabetes and Digestive and Kidney Diseases criteria for IC had a negative potassium sensitivity test. Further studies revealed only minimal improvement with known treatments [63]. Increased urothelial permeability was also found to be prevalent in detrusor overactivity and thus not specific to IC/BPS [64]. For these reasons, **potassium sensitivity testing is not recommended in the American Urological Association Interstitial Cystitis/ Bladder Pain Syndrome Guidelines** [65].

Bethanechol, a muscarinic agonist, has also been investigated in the evaluation of detrusor underactivity. Use of bethanechol to aid with postoperative urinary retention was reported as early as the 1940s. Later, the bethanechol supersensitivity test was described as part of the evaluation of a neurogenic bladder [66–68]. The test involved the instillation of 100 cc of fluid intravesically followed by administration of 2.5 mg of subcutaneous bethanechol. Repetition of fluid instillation and bethanechol administration would occur every 10 min up to three times. A positive test was indicated by an increase in the detrusor pressure by at least 15 cm H_2O at 30 min. This reflected a neurologic etiology to the detrusor dysfunction instead of a myogenic cause. Further evaluation found only moderate sensitivity (76 %) and poor specificity (50 %) of this test [69], as well as inconsistent efficacy in the treatment of an underactive bladder [70–72]. As the results of this testing would not change the management of the patient (i.e., the need for intermittent catheterization), **the use of bethanechol for bladder stimulation is no long recommended.**

More recently, edrophonium, a short-acting cholinergic agonist, has been investigated as a new provocative agent for bladder overactivity, specifically aimed for those who do not have overactivity symptoms. One small study demonstrated a response in 78 % of patients with overactive symptoms at baseline, of whom 64 % had baseline normal cystometry results [73]. Unfortunately, this study suffered from methodologic flaws (zeroing intracorporealy) and failed to show consistent subjective or objective responses to the edrophonium. **No provocative medications are used at our institution.**

Storage

The ability of the bladder to store urine is constantly assessed during cystometry. One means of assessing bladder storage is to ask the patient about their sensation of filling. More specifically, the volumes at which a patient reports his/her "first sense of bladder filling," "first desire to void," and "strong desire to void" can greatly help to characterize the patient's bladder. Further, assessing when a patient has a "strong desire to void" or significant urgency that does not abate typically defines a patient's maximal cystometric capacity.

Outside of simple bladder volume sensation, objective measures of the ability of the bladder to store urine can be expressed by means of compliance. **Compliance is the opposite of stiffness and indicates the amount of bladder wall elasticity. This is calculated as $C = \Delta V/\Delta Pdet$.**

More formally, bladder compliance is defined as the "change in volume relative to the corresponding change in the intravesical pressure" and is measured in units of mL/cm H_2O [74]. The initial proposed cutoff for low compliance was 5 mL/cm H_2O but further study demonstrated a wide range of normal among healthy subjects, likely due to the diversity in bladder volumes and most investigators currently consider normal compliance to be greater than 12.5 mL/cm H_2O [75]. Harris et al. later demonstrated that 40 mL/cm H_2O was a reasonable cutoff as the lower limit of normal [76]. This value also corresponded with a report by McGuire regarding evidence of upper tract deterioration with urethral opening pressures above 40 cm H_2O [77]. Figure 6 demonstrates a poorly compliant bladder with high pressures which would predispose a patient to obstructive nephropathy. With these findings, some have suggested that detrusor pressure may be a more useful tool for evaluating compliance changes than an actual calculated compliance value.

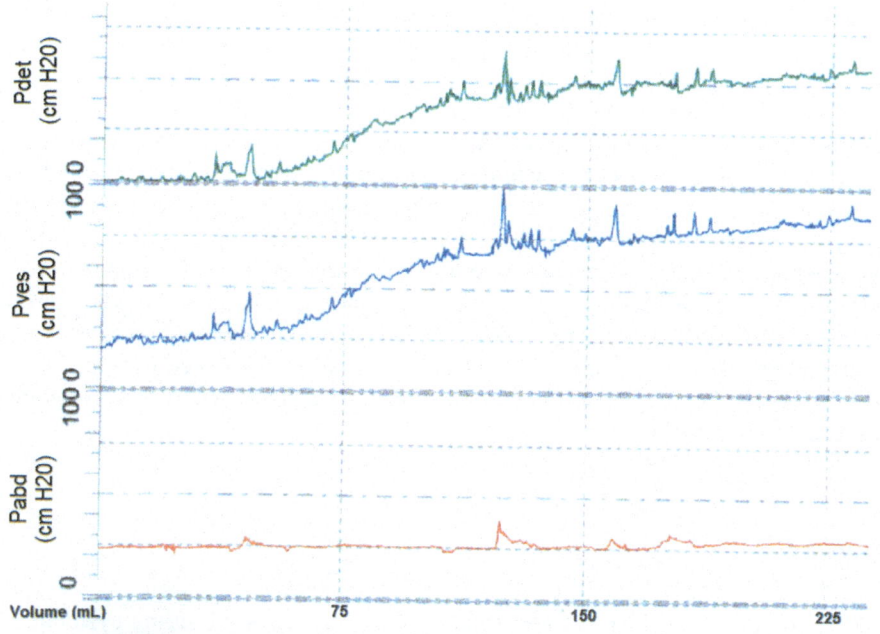

Fig. 6 Abnormal bladder compliance

Leak Point Pressure

Leak point pressure is the pressure at which a patient experiences urinary loss in the absence of a detrusor contraction during urodynamic testing. **There are two different leak point pressures that are routinely measured: the abdominal (ALPP) and the detrusor (DLPP). The abdominal leak point pressure (ALPP), is the intravesical pressure at which urine leaks due to an elevated abdominal pressure.** This is ostensibly a measure of the patient's sphincteric strength and can be used to demonstrate SUI or intrinsic sphincter deficiency. Attempts have been made to use this measure to define intrinsic sphincter deficiency as an ALPP less than 60 cm H_2O [78]. However, given that urethral hypermobility is also typically present, it is difficult to make this value an absolute cutoff. The ALPP is commonly assessed via either performance of the Valsalva maneuver (VLPP) or with a cough (CLPP). Studies have demonstrated that both maneuvers are effective in eliciting SUI but have different effects on the urethra [79]. Figure 7 demonstrates an example of a positive VLPP assessment. It has also been shown that while CLPP is typically larger than the VLPP, VLPP demonstrates less variability in provoking SUI [80, 81]. The presence of a urethral catheter has been shown to have an obstructive effect, thus leading to an exaggerated ALPP value [81]. This has thus made placement of a rectal catheter even more important. **The detrusor leak point pressure (DLPP) is defined by Abrams as the "lowest detrusor pressure at which urine leakage occurs in the absence of either a detrusor contraction or increased abdominal pressure"** [36]. This parameter is an especially important element of evaluation in those with neurogenic bladder given the known possibility for renal dysfunction and upper tract compromise with detrusor pressures >40 cm H_2O [82]. Other factors that may affect these results include the presence of pelvic organ prolapse, which can create a reservoir effect and affect abdominal pressure transmission to the urethra, patient positioning (as discussed above), and bladder volume. The recommended volume to perform this testing is half the normal cystometric capacity, typically 200–300 mL, though some studies have suggested that this capacity is too large and that testing should begin at smaller volumes (~150 mL) [83]. Other investigators utilize a voiding diary to establish the volume at which patients should undergo this testing and given the wide variations in bladder capacity, the optimal value should be determined based upon a patient's voiding diary. Videourodynamics can also be used to assess the DLPP and ALPP. **Our institution utilizes the Valsalva maneuver at a bladder volume of 200 mL and repeats this testing at 300 mL under fluoroscopy in the standing position.** In addition, if there is evidence on the pre-cystometry physical exam or during fluoroscopic evaluation of filling of pelvic organ prolapse, cystometry is repeated after performance of the voiding phase with vaginal packing in place to further characterize bladder function with proper anatomic positioning of the pelvic organs.

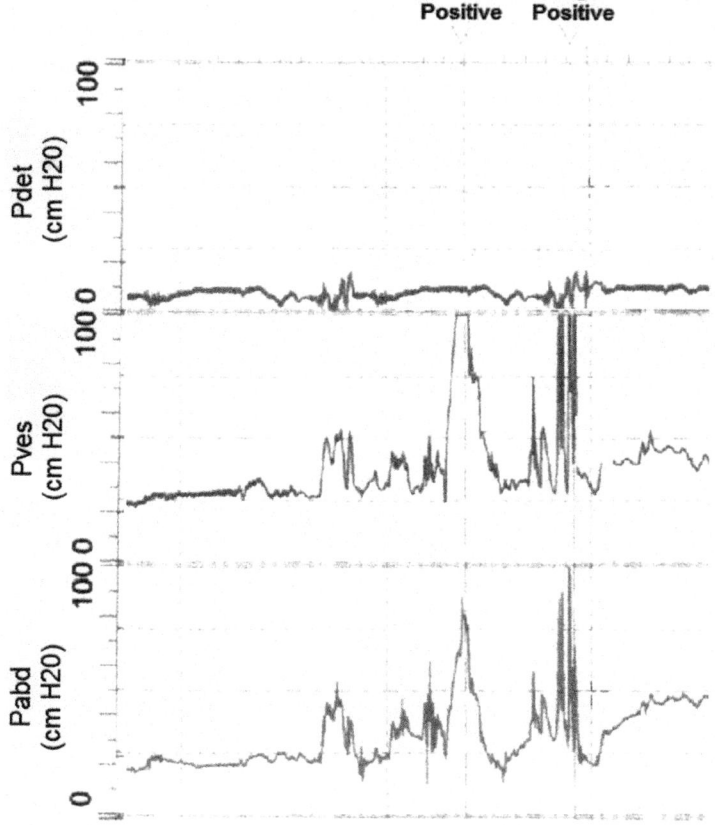

Fig. 7 A positive Valsalva leak point pressure and cough leak point pressure elicited during testing

Troubleshooting Common Problems

The most commonly encountered problem is an abnormally elevated pressure measurement, typically occurring in the rectal catheter. This is most often related to catheter positioning against the rectal wall. Thus, the first step in attempting to rectify this abnormality is to reposition the catheter by gently advancing and/or twisting the catheter so as to move it away from the intestinal wall. In the case of an abnormally elevated abdominal pressure, if repositioning proves unsuccessful, removal of <1 cc from the rectal balloon can be attempted next as overinflation of the rectal balloon can lead to elastic stretching and thus elevated pressures. If the abnormality remains, spiking the transducer or asking the patient to cough can then be performed to ensure that the problem is not due to signal transmission. Further, a cough can help to jostle an air bubble or other obstructive element from within/on the catheter. The catheters can also be inspected at this time to ensure that no kinks are present. If kinks are encountered, the obstruction can be relieved by re-taping the catheter in a different location in order to avoid any angulation to the catheter which could lead to future kinks. If the pressure remains abnormally elevated, the catheters can be disconnected from the transducers and flushed gently with ~5 mL of fluid to assess for obstruction from particulate or an air bubble. We make all attempts to avoid flushing the lines as this opens a closed system to the atmosphere, thus requiring that the lines be re-zeroed in order to ensure accurate measurements. If the pressure still does not normalize, the catheter can be exchanged for a new one given the possibility of a product defect.

Another problem that is encountered is **abnormally low pressures or non-transduction of a signal.** This usually signifies that a catheter has been pushed out and will typically occur during or after performance of the Valsalva maneuver. If the rectal catheter is pushed out, the abdominal pressure will go to zero and the detrusor pressure will be elevated and equivalent to the intravesical pressure. If this were to occur, bladder filling is paused and the rectal catheter is simply reinserted. No re-zeroing is needed as long as the transducer system/tubing remains closed to the atmosphere. If the urethral catheter is pushed out, the intravesical pressure will go to zero, thus causing the detrusor pressure to be negative and equivalent to the abdominal pressure. If this occurs, bladder filling is stopped and the catheter is replaced. A special notation is made on the graphical reporting of this event and an estimated volume lost from the filling bottle and/or bladder is recorded.

References

1. Brown M, Wicksham J. The urethral pressure profile. Br J Urol. 1969;41:211–4.
2. Gammie A, et al. International Continence Society guidelines on urodynamic equipment performance. Neurourol Urodyn. 2014;33(4):370–9.
3. Cooper MA, et al. Comparison of air-charged and water-filled urodynamic pressure measurement catheters. Neurourol Urodyn. 2011;30(3):329–34.
4. Millar HD, Baker LE. A stable ultraminiature catheter-tip pressure transducer. Med Biol Eng. 1973;11(1):86–9.
5. Asmussen M, Ulmsten U. Simultaneous urethrocystometry and urethra pressure profile measurement with a new technique. Acta Obstet Gynecol Scand. 1975;54(4):385–6.
6. Lotze PM. A comparison of external transducers and microtransducers in urodynamic studies of female patients. Curr Urol Rep. 2005;6(5):326–34.
7. Schafer W, et al. Good urodynamic practices: uroflowmetry, filling cystometry, and pressure-flow studies. Neurourol Urodyn. 2002;21(3):261–74.
8. Reynard JM, et al. The obstructive effect of a urethral catheter. J Urol. 1996;155(3):901–3.
9. Klingler HC, Madersbacher S, Schmidbauer CP. Impact of different sized catheters on pressure-flow studies in patients with benign prostatic hyperplasia. Neurourol Urodyn. 1996;15(5):473–81.
10. Baseman AG, et al. Effect of 6 F urethral catheterization on urinary flow rates during repeated pressure-flow studies in healthy female volunteers. Urology. 2002;59(6):843–6.

11. Walker RM, et al. Pressure-flow studies in the diagnosis of bladder outlet obstruction: a study comparing suprapubic and transurethral techniques. Br J Urol. 1997;79(5):693–7.
12. McCarthy TA. Validity of rectal pressure measurements as indication of intra-abdominal pressure changes during urodynamic evaluation. Urology. 1982;20(6):657–60.
13. Dall FH, et al. Biomechanical wall properties of the human rectum. A study with impedance planimetry. Gut. 1993;34(11):1581–6.
14. Dolan LM, et al. Randomized comparison of vaginal and rectal measurement of intra-abdominal pressure during subtracted dual-channel cystometry. Urology. 2005;65(6):1059–63.
15. Bhatia NN, Bergman A. Urodynamic appraisal of vaginal versus rectal pressure recordings as indication of intra-abdominal pressure changes. Urology. 1986;27(5):482–5.
16. Wall LL, Hewitt JK, Helms MJ. Are vaginal and rectal pressures equivalent approximations of one another for the purpose of performing subtracted cystometry? Obstet Gynecol. 1995;85(4):488–93.
17. Wein AJ, et al. The reproducibility and interpretation of carbon dioxide cystometry. J Urol. 1978;120(2):205–6.
18. Bracco Diagnostics Inc. (2014, October 13) *Cystografin (30 %) and Cystografin Dilute (18 %)* [Material Safety Data Sheet]. Retrieved from: http://imaging.bracco.com/sites/braccoimaging.com/files/technica_sheet_pdf/Cystografin%20and%20Cystografin%20Dilute%20SDS.pdf. Accessed 24 July 2014.
19. Aslund K, Rentzhogh L, Sandstromb G. Effects of ice cold saline and acid solution in urodynamics. In: Proceedings of the 18th Annual Meeting of the International Continence Society, Oslo, Norway. 1988.
20. Lavin JM, Hosker G, Smith ARB. Does urinary pH influence micturition desire? Neurourol Urodyn. 1997;16(5):396–7.
21. Sethia KK, Smith JC. The effect of pH and lignocaine on detrusor instability. Br J Urol. 1987;60(6):516–8.
22. Mortensen S, et al. Urodynamic implications of the differences in the viscosity of saline, urine, Urografin. In: Proceedings of the 10th Annual Meeting of the International Continence Society, Rome, Italy. 1979.
23. Hosker G, et al. A comparison of normal saline and urografin 150 for cystometry in women. In: Proceedings of the 29th Annual Meeting of the International Continence Society, Denver, Colorado. 1999.
24. Bors EH, Blinn KA. Spinal reflex activity from the vesical mucosa in paraplegic patients. AMA Arch Neurol Psychiatry. 1957;78(4):339–54.
25. Fall M, Lindstrom S, Mazieres L. Experimental aspects on the bladder cooling reflex. Neurourol Urodyn. 1987;6:228–9.
26. Lindstrom S, Mazieres L, Fall M. The bladder cooling reflex: characterization of afferent mechanism. Neurourol Urodyn. 1988;7:248–9.
27. Fall M, Lindstrom S, Mazieres L. A bladder-to-bladder cooling reflex in the cat. J Physiol. 1990;427:281–300.
28. Lindstrom S, Mazieres L. Effect of menthol on the bladder cooling reflex in the cat. Acta Physiol Scand. 1991;141(1):1–10.
29. Hellstrom PA, et al. The bladder cooling test for urodynamic assessment: analysis of 400 examinations. Br J Urol. 1991;67(3):275–9.
30. Geirsson G, Lindstrom S, Fall M. The bladder cooling reflex in man–characteristics and sensitivity to temperature. Br J Urol. 1993;71(6):675–80.
31. Ronzoni G, et al. The ice-water test in the diagnosis and treatment of the neurogenic bladder. Br J Urol. 1997;79(5):698–701.
32. Mazières L, Jiang C, Lindström S. The C fibre reflex of the cat urinary bladder. J Physiol. 1998;513(2):531–41.
33. Geirsson G, Lindström S, Fall M. The bladder cooling reflex and the use of cooling as stimulus to the lower urinary tract. J Urol. 1999;162(6):1890–6.
34. McDonald DF, Murphy GP. Quantitative studies of perception of thermal stimuli in the normal and neurogenic urinary bladder. J Appl Physiol. 1959;14(2):204–6.

35. Stohrer M, et al. The standardization of terminology in neurogenic lower urinary tract dysfunction: with suggestions for diagnostic procedures. International Continence Society Standardization Committee. Neurourol Urodyn. 1999;18(2):139–58.
36. Abrams P, et al. The standardisation of terminology of lower urinary tract function: report from the Standardisation Sub-committee of the International Continence Society. Neurourol Urodyn. 2002;21(2):167–78.
37. Klevmark B. Natural pressure-volume curves and conventional cystometry. Scand J Urol Nephrol Suppl. 1999;201:1–4.
38. Stöhrer M, et al. EAU guidelines on neurogenic lower urinary tract dysfunction. Eur Urol. 2009;56(1):81–8.
39. Sørensen S, et al. Changes in bladder volumes with repetition of water cystometry. Urol Res. 1984;12(4):205–8.
40. Cass A, Ward B, Markland C. Comparison of slow and rapid fill cystometry using liquid and air. J Urol. 1970;104(1):104.
41. Nordling J, Walter S. Repeated, rapid fill CO_2-cystometry. Urol Res. 1977;5(3):117–22.
42. Jarvis G, et al. An assessment of urodynamic examination in incontinent women. Br J Obstet Gynaecol. 1980;87(10):893–6.
43. Versi E, et al. Symptoms analysis for the diagnosis of genuine stress incontinence. Br J Obstet Gynaecol. 1991;98(8):815–9.
44. Scotti RJ, Myers DL. A comparison of the cough stress test and single-channel cystometry with multichannel urodynamic evaluation in genuine stress incontinence. Obstet Gynecol. 1993;81(3):430–3.
45. Swift SE, Ostergard DR. Evaluation of current urodynamic testing methods in the diagnosis of genuine stress incontinence. Obstet Gynecol. 1995;86(1):85–91.
46. Richardson DA. Value of the cough pressure profile in the evaluation of patients with stress incontinence. Am J Obstet Gynecol. 1986;155(4):808–11.
47. Mayer R, et al. Handwashing in the cystometric evaluation of detrusor instability. Neurourol Urodyn. 1991;10(6):563–9.
48. Radley SC, et al. Conventional and ambulatory urodynamic findings in women with symptoms suggestive of bladder overactivity. J Urol. 2001;166(6):2253–8.
49. Sand PK, Hill RC, Ostergard DR. Supine urethroscopic and standing cystometry as screening methods for the detection of detrusor instability. Obstet Gynecol. 1987;70(1):57–60.
50. Andersen JT, Bradley WE. Postural detrusor hyperreflexia. J Urol. 1976;116(2):228–30.
51. Mayo ME. Detrusor hyperreflexia: the effect of posture and pelvic floor activity. J Urol. 1978;119(5):635–8.
52. Godec C, Cass A. Cystometric variations during postural changes and functional electrical stimulation of the pelvic floor muscles. J Urol. 1980;123(5):722–5.
53. Awad S, McGinnis R. Factors that influence the incidence of detrusor instability in women. J Urol. 1983;130(1):114–5.
54. Arunkalaivanan A, Mahomoud S, Howell M. Does posture affect cystometric parameters and diagnoses? Int Urogynecol J. 2004;15(6):422–4.
55. Ramsden PD, et al. The unstable bladder–fact or artefact? Br J Urol. 1977;49(7):633–9.
56. Lockhart J, et al. Urodynamics in women with stress and urge incontinence. Urology. 1982;20(3):333–6.
57. Choe JM, Gallo ML, Staskin DR. A provocative maneuver to elicit cystometric instability: measuring instability at maximum infusion. J Urol. 1999;161(5):1541–4.
58. Eastwood H. Postural influences on urinary incontinence in the elderly. Gerontology. 1986;32(4):207–10.
59. Al-Hayek S, Belal M, Abrams P. Does the patient's position influence the detection of detrusor overactivity? Neurourol Urodyn. 2008;27(4):279–86.
60. Parsons CL, et al. The role of urinary potassium in the pathogenesis and diagnosis of interstitial cystitis. J Urol. 1998;159(6):1862–6. discussion 1866-7.
61. Bernie JE, et al. The intravesical potassium sensitivity test and urodynamics: implications in a large cohort of patients with lower urinary tract symptoms. J Urol. 2001;166(1):158–61.

62. Daha LK, et al. Comparative assessment of maximal bladder capacity, 0.9 % NaCl versus 0.2 M KCl, for the diagnosis of interstitial cystitis: a prospective controlled study. J Urol. 2003;170(3):807–9.
63. Teichman JM, Nielsen-Omeis BJ. Potassium leak test predicts outcome in interstitial cystitis. J Urol. 1999;161(6):1791–4. discussion 1794–6.
64. Philip J, Willmott S, Irwin P. Interstitial cystitis versus detrusor overactivity: a comparative, randomized, controlled study of cystometry using saline and 0.3 M potassium chloride. J Urol. 2006;175(2):566–70. discussion 570–1.
65. Hanno PM, et al. AUA guideline for the diagnosis and treatment of interstitial cystitis/bladder pain syndrome. J Urol. 2011;185(6):2162–70.
66. Diokno AC, Koppenhoefer R. Bethanechol chloride in neurogenic bladder dysfunction. Urology. 1976;8(5):455–8.
67. Diokno AC, Lapides J. Action of oral and parenteral bethanechol on decompensated bladder. Urology. 1977;10(1):23–4.
68. Lapides J, et al. A new method for diagnosing the neurogenic bladder. Med Bull (Ann Arbor). 1962;28:166–80.
69. Blaivas JG, et al. Failure of bethanechol denervation supersensitivity as a diagnostic aid. J Urol. 1980;123(2):199–201.
70. Wein A, et al. The effects of bethanechol chloride on urodynamic parameters in normal women and in women with significant residual urine volumes. J Urol. 1980;124(3):397–9.
71. Barrett D. The effect of oral bethanechol chloride on voiding in female patients with excessive residual urine: a randomized double-blind study. J Urol. 1981;126(5):640–2.
72. Wein AJ, et al. The effect of oral bethanechol chloride on the cystometrogram of the normal male adult. J Urol. 1978;120(3):330–1.
73. Yossepowitch O, et al. The effect of cholinergic enhancement during filling cystometry: can edrophonium chloride be used as a provocative test for overactive bladder? J Urol. 2001;165(5):1441–5.
74. Wein AJ, Kavoussi LR, Campbell MF. Campbell-Walsh urology. Editor-in-chief, Alan J. Wein [Kavoussi LR, et al., editors]. 10th ed. Philadelphia, PA: Elsevier Saunders; 2012.
75. Toppercer A, Tetreault JP. Compliance of the bladder: an attempt to establish normal values. Urology. 1979;14(2):204–5.
76. Harris RL, et al. Bladder compliance in neurologically intact women. Neurourol Urodyn. 1996;15(5):483–8.
77. McGuire E, et al. Prognostic value of urodynamic testing in myelodysplastic patients. J Urol. 1981;126(2):205–9.
78. McGuire E, et al. Clinical assessment of urethral sphincter function. J Urol. 1993;150(5 Pt 1):1452–4.
79. McGuire EJ, Cespedes RD, O'Connell HE. Leak-point pressures. Urol Clin North Am. 1996;23(2):253–62.
80. Kuo HC. Videourodynamic analysis of the relationship of Valsalva and cough leak point pressures in women with stress urinary incontinence. Urology. 2003;61(3):544–8. discussion 548–9.
81. Bump RC, et al. Valsalva leak point pressures in women with genuine stress incontinence: reproducibility, effect of catheter caliber, and correlations with other measures of urethral resistance. Continence Program for Women Research Group. Am J Obstet Gynecol. 1995;173(2):551–7.
82. Wang S, McGuire E, Bloom D. A bladder pressure management system for myelodysplasia–clinical outcome. J Urol. 1988;140(6):1499–502.
83. Miklos JR, Sze EH, Karram MM. A critical appraisal of the methods of measuring leak-point pressures in women with stress incontinence. Obstet Gynecol. 1995;86(3):349–52.

The Pressure Flow Study

Kirk M. Anderson and David A. Hadley

Introduction

The best method of analyzing voiding function quantitatively is the pressure-flow study (PFS) of micturition, with simultaneous recording of abdominal, intravesical, and detrusor pressures, volume voided and flow rate. Direct inspection of the raw pressure and flow data before, during, and at the end of micturition is essential because it allows artifacts and equipment limitations to be recognized and eliminated. The flow of urine depends on the generation of a bladder power that can overcome the resistance of a dynamic outlet. In the absence of detrusor and bladder outlet abnormality, pressure-flow tracings follow a predictable pattern. Once micturition is initiated, detrusor pressure increases until the opening pressure is reached at which point urine flow begins. Maximum urine flow is attained during contraction and as the bladder volume decreases, detrusor pressure and flow rate decrease until the bladder is empty (Table 1).

K.M. Anderson, M.D. (✉)
Department of Urology, University of Colorado, 2631 East 17th Ave., M/S-C-319, Aurora, CO 80045, USA
e-mail: kirk.anderson@ucdenver.edu

D.A. Hadley, M.D.
Loma Linda Urology, Loma Linda University Medical Center, 11234 Anderson St., Room A560, Loma Linda, CA 92354, USA
e-mail: davidhadley@llu.edu

Table 1 Key terms and definitions

Term	Definition
Maximum flow rate (Q_{max})	The maximum measured value of the flow rate
Maximum pressure ($p_{abd.max}$, $p_{ves.max}$, $p_{det.max}$)	The maximum value of the pressure measured during a pressure-flow study
Pressure at maximum flow ($p_{abd.Qmax}$, $p_{ves.Qmax}$, $p_{det.Qmax}$)	The pressure recorded at maximum measured flow rate. If the same maximum value is attained more than once or if it is sustained for a period of time, then the point of maximum flow is taken to be where the detrusor pressure has its lowest value for this flow rate; abdominal, intravesical, and detrusor pressures at maximum flow are all read at the same point
Opening pressure ($p_{abd.open}$, $p_{ves.open}$, $p_{det.open}$)	The pressure recorded at the onset of measured flow
Closing pressure ($p_{abd.clos}$, $p_{ves.clos}$, $p_{det.clos}$)	The pressure recorded at the end of measured flow
Minimum voiding pressure ($p_{det.min.void}$)	The minimum pressure during measurable flow. It may be, but is not necessarily, equal to the opening pressure or the closing pressure

From Griffiths D, Hoefner K, van Mastrigt R, Rollema HJ, Spangberg A, Gleason D (1998) Standardization of terminology of lower urinary tract function: pressure-flow studies of voiding, urethral resistance, and urethral obstructions. Neurology and Urodynamics, with permission of John Wiley & Sons

Introduction to Nomograms

While nomograms are discussed in detail elsewhere (chapter "Nomograms") a brief discussion in this section is pertinent. Mathematical descriptions and relationships that can be used to characterize voiding and degrees of obstruction have evolved significantly. Initially, the relationship between pressure and flow was based on the presupposition that the bladder and urethra functioned under basic rigid tube and spherical hydrodynamic principles [1]. Under this model of a rigid pipe, for a given pressure (p) the cross sectional area (A) of the tube determines flow rate (Q).

$$Q = A \sqrt{2p_{det}}$$

This is a simplified variation of Bernoulli's equation [2]. However, a large assumption made in this simple rigid model is that all pressure is converted to flow velocity. This model fails to take into consideration the distensibility, or elasticity of the urethra. In the 1960s a distensible and collapsible system was described where pressure is required to distend the urethral lumen [3, 4]. Since even with a fully relaxed pelvic floor, the urethra will still be collapsed. Pressure-energy is then consumed during this process of opening the urethra during voiding and is not converted to flow. **This "energy", or elasticity, has been termed the minimal urethral opening pressure (p_{muo}) or now the minimum voiding pressure ($p_{det.min.void}$) in**

International Continence Society (ICS) terminology [5]. So now flow is dependent on the cross sectional area and the urethral opening pressure, which then modifies the equation:

$$Q = A\sqrt{2(p_{det} - p_{det.min.void})}$$

According to this principle, the flow of urine will only occur when intrinsic bladder pressure equals the intrinsic urethral pressure [2]. The $p_{det.min.void}$, is very important for diagnosing obstruction, as it is the minimum voiding pressure documented during measurable flow and may differ from the "opening pressure" or "closing pressure" [5]. It is typically measured at the end of voiding, with strong consideration to both equipment flow delay and the draining of the distal urethra (approximately the last 5–10 mL and/or flow rate less than 2 mL/s). This number should always be read on the original tracings and clinicians should avoid the temptation to allow the software to read these without validation by the physician [6].

Although it was recognized that the urethra was not a rigid pipe, it was still initially assumed that once the urethra was opened, it could be treated as a rigid structure. This assumption was based on the interpretation of fluoroscopic images that showed that the urethra did not appear to have any major changes in size and/or shape during voiding. However, even when the shape is unchanged, the distensible tube is still fundamentally different from a rigid one, because the fluid is still under the elastic laws of the urethral wall [2]. From this, it follows that these elastic laws, which vary in significance along the urethra, control the flow rate. **So for a fixed pressure, the maximum flow rate is controlled by the area with the combination of least elasticity and smallest lumen of the urethra, termed the flow controlling zone (FCZ)** [7]. **The FCZ is the area of highest pressure within the urethra, and not necessarily the area with the smallest lumen** [8].

As summarized by Schaefer, "...an important difference between flow in a rigid and an elastic outlet is related to the flow controlling zone. In a rigid system the whole length of the bladder outlet from the bladder neck to the meatus contributes to the fluid energy losses, and the size of the meatal exit area controls the flow rate. In an elastically distensible system the pressure/flow rate relation is governed by the size and elasticity of a flow rate controlling zone, which in general is not the exit area. Physiologically, this zone is located at the genitourinary diaphragm, so that only the fluid energy losses upstream from there can affect the flow rate, and the meatus controls only the exit velocity of the urinary stream" [2].

In addition, a few properties are considered and have been proven to be negligible to simplify the above equations: flow is steady through a constant cross-sectional area, fluid viscosity and other energy losses are negligible, and outlet pressure is the same near the beginning and end of voiding. If negligible, the relationship between pressure and flow is controlled by the elasticity ($p_{det.min.void}$) and the urethral cross sectional area (A) as previously shown. In men, this is at the junction of the prostatic and membranous urethra, while in women, this is at the mid-point of the urethra [8]. Men with a longer urethra should have statistically significant higher energy losses according to the above hydrodynamic principles. But the FCZ is close to bladder and controls the flow rate. The urethra above this area does result in energy losses but given its relatively short length, it is more akin to the length of the female urethra, and these short distances have proven negligible and are not included in the above equations [2]. The exact equations and explanations for this are beyond the scope of this chapter.

With this now better understood, Griffiths set out to determine and measure the properties of the this flow controlling zone during voiding. For a known urethra, he did near continuous plotting of corresponding Q's and p's during an entire void, and plotted this on a detrusor pressure-flow rate graph. The relationship representing the detrusor pressure needed to propel urine through a urethra at a particular flow rate he termed the urethral resistance relation (URR), and it is dependent only on the urethral mechanical properties [8]. In other words, for a urethra with constant mechanical properties, as the flow rate increases, so must the intrinsic bladder pressure.

Unfortunately, this required finding multiple points to plot that were all affected significantly by the inherent flow delay and other artifacts in urodynamics. Today, this can be plotted as a continuous line on a pressure-flow chart, but initially required multiple individual points that were then connected by a line. The passive urethral resistance relation (PURR) was described by Schafer in the 1980s and was the first attempt to simplify the URR [2, 9]. The PURR is fundamentally based on Griffith's work of urethral resistance relation (URR), but describes the relationship between pressure and flow during the period of lowest urethral resistance. This requires a computer program to calculate the curve based on the continuous pressure flow graph in attempt to simulate the pressure-flow relationship if complete urethral relaxation, or the largest possible A, occurred during the entire void (Fig. 1). The purpose of this is to most closely evaluate the true morphology of a particular bladder outlet, in order to evaluate for inherent obstruction. Of note, deviations from the PURR are considered to be from the variable contractions of the external sphincter during voiding (active) or slow distensibility of the urethra (passive) [10].

Subsequently, Schaefer noted that the curve of the PURR was of only secondary importance clinically and required a computer to calculate, so to further simplify, the PURR curve was traded for a straight line, and termed the linear PURR or LinPURR (Fig. 1). The two points at the ends of this line are the $p_{det.min.void}$, or the lowest pressure where flow starts or stops, and $p_{det.Qmax}$ [6]. From these lines the Schaeffer nomogram was derived. In separate but similar work, Abrams and Griffiths developed the bladder outlet obstruction index (BOOI), previously referred to as the AG number, which was initially derived from pressure-flow studies in 117 men >55 years old with suspected prostatic obstruction [11]. The equation was derived from the line dividing the obstructed from the equivocal range on a scatter plot of the Abrams-Griffiths study:

$$\mathbf{BOOI} = p_{det.Qmax} \quad 2Q_{max}$$

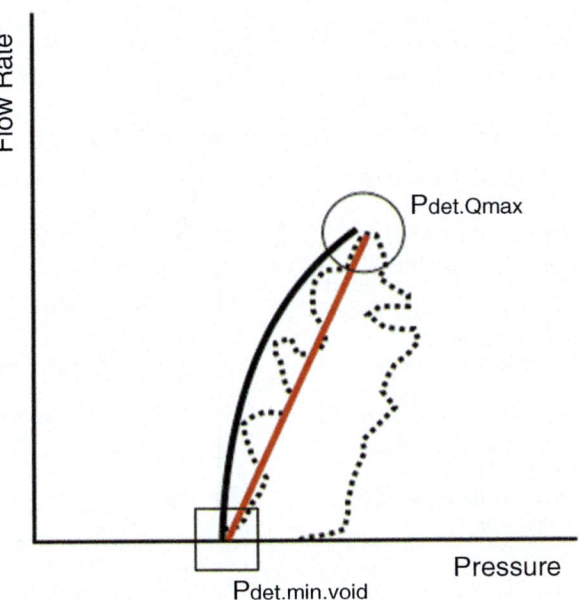

Fig. 1 Pressure-Flow graph on a micturition. *Dotted line* represents a continuous URR during the void. *Black line* represents the PURR that is the idealized pressure-flow plot of the urethra in a completely relaxed state. It is computer derived from analyzing a continuous URR. *Red line* represents the linear PURR which connects the $p_{det.Qmax}$ and the pdet.min.void [6]

where 2 is the slope of the line. **This equation became the basis for the ICS nomogram in 1997 [5], and cut off values gleaned from prior works were established**:

Obstruction—BOOI greater than 40
Equivocal—BOOI 20–40
Unobstructed—BOOI less than 20

It should be noted that to make a diagnosis of bladder obstruction (BOOI>40) p_{det} must be at least be 40 cm H_2O.

The dynamics of micturition involve both the bladder outlet and detrusor function and equations like the BOOI formula does not take into account bladder contractility. Shafer described the detrusor muscle as the source of mechanical power for voiding and the bladder outlet as a physical entity that dissipates this power (Pext) in the form of flow rate and pressure during voiding [2, 9].

$$Pext = p \times Q$$

The detrusor provides the power but the outlet determines how this is split into pressure or flow rate. Therefore, the flow rate and detrusor pressure have an inverse relationship, for a given power of external voiding (Pext), the product of the two must be constant. A high flow suggests a low pressure (normal voiding) and a low flow suggests a high pressure (obstruction). This is graphically represented by the Hill equation and the hyperbolic curve shows the low pressure-high flow and high pressure-low flow voiding relationship (Fig. 2). This represents the bladder-output

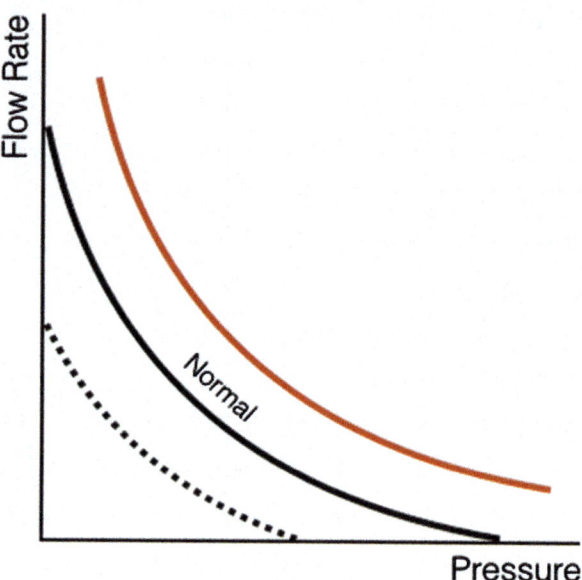

Fig. 2 The bladder output relation, showing the relationship between high pressure-low flow and low pressure-high flow. This *hyperbolic line* is for a given detrusor power. It can shift up and to the *right* (*red line*) with increasing volume that maximizes the prestretched length of the muscle fibers thus increasing the available power. In this instance both the pressure and flow will increase. Conversely it can shift down and to the *left* (*dotted line*) with decreased filling or detrusor decompensation [6, 12]

relation (BOR) and like other muscles, the detrusor has a fundamental relation between the force of contraction (detrusor pressure) and the speed of shortening of the muscle (flow rate) [12]. This inverse relation is an inherent myogenic trait and it is important to recognize that this can only apply when there is a "normal" or given, detrusor muscle power. The curve is not fixed and power can change for a particular detrusor system. Increasing the prestreched length of muscle fibers (to a point) by increasing bladder filling volume increases power and higher flow is possible. And correspondingly, decreasing bladder volume or detrusor decompensation will decrease power. Therefore, it is not only the bladder outlet (FCZ) but also the detrusor power-volume relation that determines peak flow [6]. The Bladder Contractility Index (BCI), discussed further in the following section, is derived from the work by Schafer and categorizes men according to strength of bladder contractility.

This developing understanding of the hydrodynamics of the bladder and bladder outlet resulted in the development of nomograms to objectively categorize male patients with bothersome lower urinary tract symptoms. When the BCI and BOOI nomograms are overlaid, a data point can be categorized in one of nine zones ranging from no obstruction with good contractility to obstruction with weak contractility. These are reviewed in further detail in chapter "Nomograms". The BOOI and BCI are easy to perform calculations that can help categorize patients according to the results of pressure-flow studies.

In the absence of outlet obstruction or neurologic dysfunction, the voiding phase of urodynamic measurements follows an expected pattern. Once volitional voiding is initiated, the detrusor begins to contract. The pressure generated prior to commencement of urine flow is the pre-micturition pressure and is broadly categorized as an isovolumetric contraction, a contraction that occurs at a consistent volume.

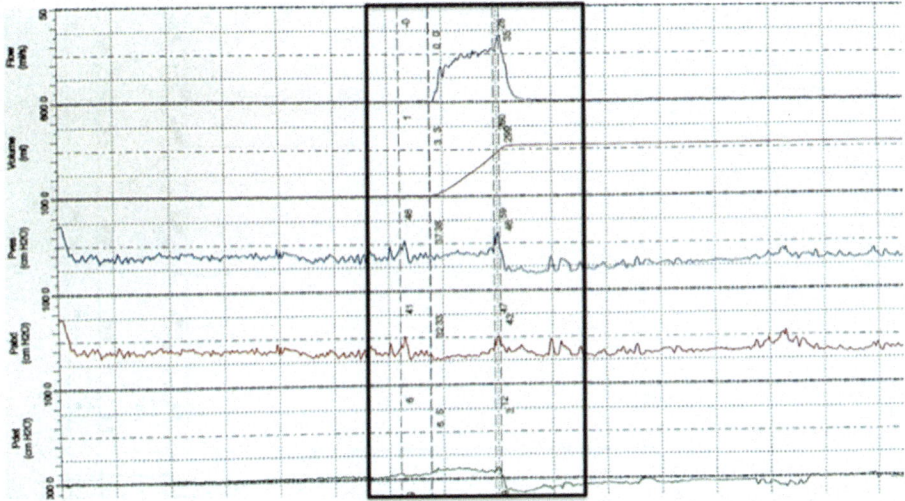

Fig. 3 Low pressure-high flow pattern seen in normal voiding

The abdominal and intravesical pressures at the onset of flow are recorded and the difference between these values represents the opening detrusor pressure. As detrusor pressure increases, the urethra distends (increasing A of the FCZ) and subsequently flow rate increases to its maximum rate, Q_{max}. Detrusor pressure at Q_{max} is also recorded as this is used in identifying conditions of obstruction as discussed previously. As the bladder empties, pressure and flow decrease. The closing pressure, the pressure at which flow stops, is recorded and the voiding phase is complete (Fig. 3).

Bladder Outlet Obstruction in Males

Typically, a Q_{max} of less than 10 mL/s has been used as the cutoff to suggest obstruction in men, as this would suggest a high pressure and therefore likely obstruction. **Decreased flow rate by itself may be indicative of either outflow obstruction or impaired bladder contractility (or a combination of the two) with both the false negative and false positive rates of Q_{max} having been reported as high as 25 %** [13].

The index male patient with lower urinary tract symptoms (LUTS) has been described as middle-aged or elderly with bothersome symptoms of storage and/or voiding consisting of frequency, urgency, nocturia, as well as hesitancy, weak stream, and feeling of incomplete emptying. Unfortunately bother, prostate size, and urodynamic proven urinary obstruction are not always well correlated. Therefore it is not always benign prostatic obstruction (BPO) caused by benign prostatic enlargement (BPE) causing LUTS in men [14]. In the presence of normal detrusor function, pressure-flow tracings of men with bladder outlet obstruction (BOO) appear as a high-pressure, low-flow pattern (Fig. 4).

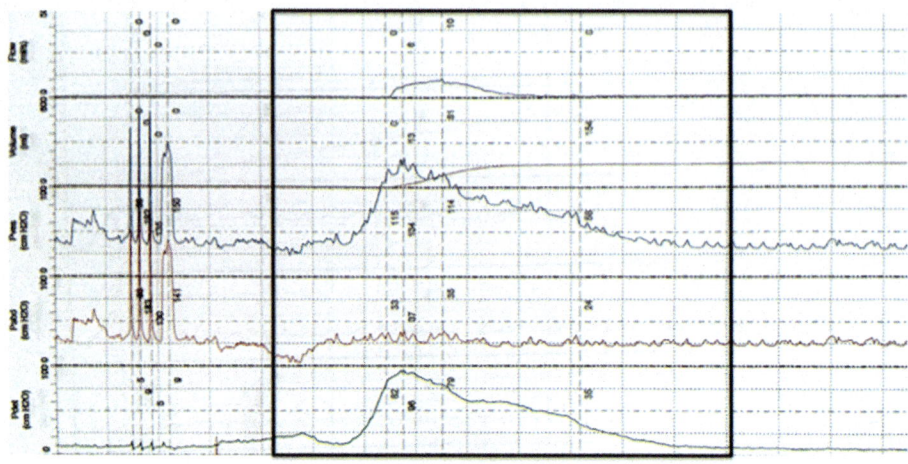

Fig. 4 High pressure-low flow pattern of obstructed voiding

The bladder outlet function is defined by two parameters (see chapter "Nomograms"): 1) opening pressure, reflecting distensibility of the tube, and 2) the cross-sectional area (A) at the FCZ. When there is an obstruction, however, the obstruction itself may take over the role of the FCZ. In BPO, higher pressure is required to open the urethra and initiate urinary flow, requiring a higher $p_{det.min.void}$, due to the prostatic urethra's reduced distensibility. However, once open and throughout voiding, the ratio of pressure to flow becomes more similar to an unobstructed system (Fig. 5). This has been described as compressive PURR, which typically raises the opening pressure but has no major changes in the P-Q curve. This occurs rarely as an isolated abnormality, but is the more pronounced effect in BPO. In contrast, constrictive PURR occurs in conditions such as urethral stricture disease, where the P-Q curve is likely to appear flat secondary to the effective smaller and fixed cross-sectional area of the diseased tissue. In this scenario, the $p_{det.min.void}$ remains unchanged, as the urethral distensibility is unchanged. However increases in pressure correspond with only small increases in flow, due to the small and fixed A of the FCZ, resulting in a flat PURR curve. Patients with bladder outlet obstruction typically have a combination of both constrictive and compressive patterns [10]. The constrictive factor becomes more significant as the grade of BPO increases. This can be seen on the Schaefer nomogram where the boundary lines become progressively flatter as the obstruction grade increases (see chapter "Nomograms") [15]. Of note, as the total power, or energy, developed by the detrusor during a single contraction cycle is limited, this larger $p_{det.min.void}$ explains why increased residual urine volumes are more commonly seen in compressive obstructions but are rare in constrictive obstructions.

Although the PFS is useful to diagnose obstruction, how does this relate clinically to patients and outcomes? Javle et al. initially showed urodynamic grading of

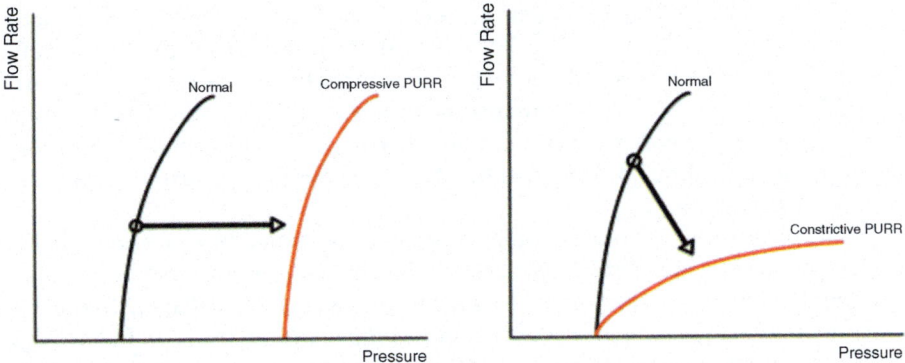

Fig. 5 A purely compressive obstruction raises the $p_{det.min.void}$ only. The pressure-flow relationship is then relatively unchanged with any increases. A purely constrictive obstruction has the same $p_{det.min.void}$ but with a flat curve because the A of the FCZ is reduced and not elastic [6]

obstruction and detrusor contractility predicted treatment outcome after prostatectomy (TURP) with a sensitivity of 87 %, specificity of 93 %, and positive predictive value of 95 % based on IPSS, flow rate, PVR, and pressure flow studies [16]. In 74 patients, Gotoh et al., slightly modified Schafer's nomogram and reported that patients with strong detrusor contractility and unequivocal obstruction on pressure-flow analysis had the best surgical outcomes subjectively and objectively. However, the majority of their patients diagnosed as having minimal obstruction and weak detrusors also benefited from relief of their obstruction [17]. In an even larger study with 253 patients, Rodrigues et al. used seven groups of obstruction to analyze their outcomes. Their results showed a clear relationship with clinical outcome and subjective satisfaction with increasing obstruction grade. In other words, the higher the obstruction, the greater the clinical benefit compared to those with little or no obstruction. Furthermore, in their analysis the non-obstructed patients did not have any clinical or subjective improvement after transurethral prostatic resection [18]. **Weak bladder contractility, equivocal or absent obstruction, and detrusor overactivity are considered to be ominous signs on PFS with worse outcomes as described in these multiple studies.**

BOO in Females

The nomograms and definitions discussed above were developed using data from male populations and do not apply to women [9]. The studies that established these findings were derived from extensively studying patients with a unique and highly prevalent condition, BPE, which does not occur in women. Also, it has been well established in other studies that women typically void at lower detrusor pressures than men. Some women are able to void solely by just relaxing their pelvic floor musculature while others may perform valsalva voiding [19].

Incidence rates of bladder outlet obstruction vary widely among symptomatic women with a range from 2.7 % to 34 % [9, 19]. **Anatomic abnormalities resulting in obstruction in women include previous incontinence surgery, pelvic surgery, high-grade pelvic organ prolapse, or urethral pathology, such as stricture, neoplasm, diverticulum, or cyst. Functional obstruction abnormalities include: dysfunctional voiding, detrusor sphincter dyssynergia, or primary bladder neck obstruction** [20].

While obstruction or voiding complaints are less common than storage or irritative symptoms in women, the importance of the voiding phase in women cannot be ignored. Voiding complaints in women include: straining to void, having to stand to void, intermittency, suprapubic pressure, or incomplete emptying [20]. In one large study, the results of cystometrogram (CMG) alone were compared to results of CMG and PFS in women with LUTS. PFS were found to have relevant information in 33 % of women and of those, 70 % had a normal CMG [21]. This is also confirmed by two large studies showing a prevalence of 5.2–19.5 % of women with voiding complaints [22, 23]. Although the definition for BOO in women is not yet well defined as it is in men, the concept of a high pressure and low flow voiding as a measure of obstruction prevails. Three predominant thoughts have been used in attempts to further define BOO in women [9, 19].

First, Chassagne et al. proposed cutoff criteria for voiding pressure and flow rate. In this and subsequent studies, the authors refined and calculated the values suggesting obstruction to $Q_{max} < 12$ or $p_{det.Qmax} > 25$ when comparing 169 clinically obstructed patients to controls [24]. While meeting both criteria was highly suggestive of obstruction, even the presence of just one abnormal parameter may be indicative of obstruction. A second definition, from Nitti et al., used videourodynamics for radiographic evidence of obstruction along with a sustained detrusor contraction [25]. No numeric values were used for strict pressure-flow criteria as specific cutoff values lacked specificity in their analysis. Please see chapter "The Use of Fluoroscopy" for further information on videourodynamics. Third, Blaivas and Groutz created a nomogram based on the on their database of 600 urodynamic patients [26]. Qualification of obstruction included at least one of the following: free $Q_{max} < 12$ mL/s and $p_{det.max} > 20$ cm H_2O in pressure-flow studies, obvious radiographic obstruction with sustained detrusor contraction of > 20 cm H_2O, urinary retention, or the inability to void with a catheter and a sustained detrusor contraction of >20 cm H_2O. Using cluster analysis, a four-zone nomogram was developed ranging from no to severe obstruction. (Please see chapter "Nomograms".) Modifications to their nomogram include using a non-invasive flow rate to the avoid the effects of a transurethral catheter and $p_{det.max}$ instead of $p_{det.Qmax}$ in order to evaluate retention patients in the nomogram [27].

Given the wide range of conditions that cause female BOO and lack of intervention outcomes, pressure flow analysis is not as standardized as it is in men [15, 19]. Therefore, a diagnosis of obstruction is supported when a combination of history, physical, PVR, uroflow and/or videourodynamics are highly suggestive of a voiding abnormality [20].

Underactive Detrusor Contraction and Valsalva Voiding

Two voiding states were discussed above; high flow-low pressure seen with normal voiding and low flow-high pressure characteristic of obstruction. A third urodynamic finding is low-pressure, low-flow voiding that is typical of impaired detrusor contractility. So low flow rate can be present with either high or low detrusor pressures, and therefore is insufficient to differentiate between obstruction and impaired contractility. Additionally, elevated post-void residual as well as symptoms of hesitancy, straining to void, and slow stream can be present in both outlet obstruction and detrusor underactivity. Currently, differentiation between obstruction and impaired bladder contractility in patients with low-flow can only be determined by simultaneous measurement of detrusor pressure and flow rate during voiding.

Low amplitude, poorly sustained detrusor contraction and low flow are typical of detrusor underactivity on urodynamics measurements (Fig. 6). Multiple etiologies exist for detrusor underactivity that can represent disruption of the neurogenic, myogenic, or a combination of these components. Common neurogenic etiologies include Parkinson's disease, multiple sclerosis, spinal cord injury, and iatrogenic insult to nerves during pelvic surgery. Myogenic changes are seen in patients with bladder outlet obstruction, diabetes, and age related changes.

Detrusor underactivity (DU), as defined by the ICS, is a detrusor contraction of reduced strength and/or duration, resulting in prolonged bladder emptying, and/or failure to achieve complete bladder emptying within a normal time span. Currently, there is no clear consensus on what a normal strength or duration is. Commonly used criteria are $p_{det.Qmax}$ <30–45 cm H$_2$O with

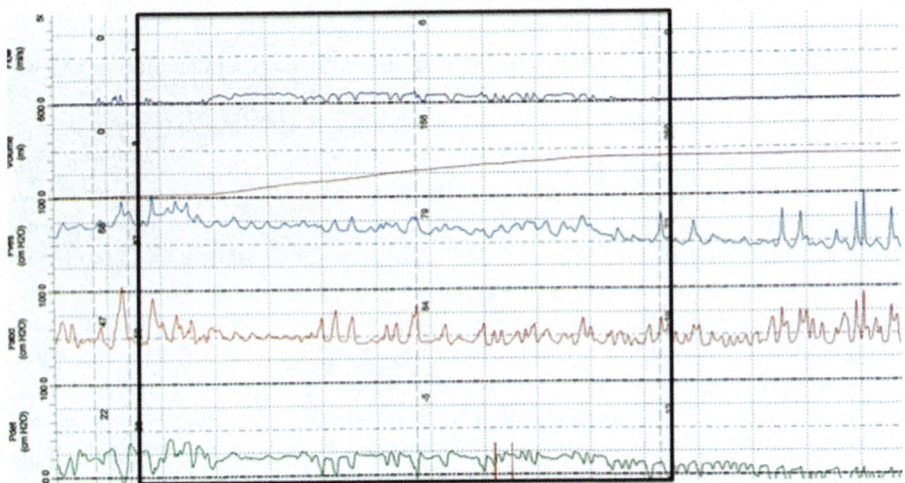

Fig. 6 Low pressure-low flow prolonged voiding pattern characteristic of detrusor underactivity

$Q_{max} < 10\text{–}15$ mL/s [28]. Additionally, the BCI was developed to objectify bladder contractility. This is based on the analysis of LinPURR from men with varying degrees of obstruction [29]. From this, three categories were established based on the following equation and are represented by the bladder contractility nomogram [30].

$$BCI = p_{det.Qmax} + 5Q_{max}$$

Strong—BCI greater than 150
Normal—BCI 100–150
Weak—BCI less than 100
Acontractile—complete absence of detrusor contraction

However, the BCI has also not been widely accepted or validated as confirmatory evidence of DU. Care should be taken during pressure-flow studies to differentiate between: inability to void due to extrinsic factors during testing vs. true detrusor acontractility. A careful history can help differentiate this.

Detrusor underactivity is estimated to be present in 10–20 % of men who present with lower urinary tract symptoms and low flow [28]. Identifying detrusor underactivity in the presence of bladder outlet obstruction can be challenging in certain patients. Bladder contractility index, as described above, can be calculated, however certain limitations exist. The calculation should be done manually to correctly identify the appropriate values, as tracing artifacts and equipment limitations will not be recognized by computer software programs. In addition to the BCI, the Watt Factor (WF) can also be calculated to objectively estimate detrusor contractility. The WF is a complex formula that is derived from consideration of the bladder volume at each point of micturition, contraction speed, and detrusor pressure during voiding. It is unknown whether using the maximum WF or the WF at maximum urine flow rate better estimates detrusor strength. Current expert opinion suggests that a maximum WF of <7 W/m^2 may indicate detrusor underactivity [19]. Currently, WF is of limited clinical utility due to the complexity of obtaining data for calculation as well as the relative lack of published data validating its clinical merit.

There is debate whether surgical treatment for suspected outlet obstruction provides benefit to men with detrusor underactivity. In a retrospective review, men with DU treated with transurethral resection of the prostate (TURP) were compared to a matched controlled group with DU who did not undergo TURP. At a mean follow-up of 11.3 years, the 16 men treated with TURP showed no statistically significant difference in symptoms of reduced stream, hesitancy, straining, frequency, post-void residual volume, or voided volume compared to the 44 mean who did not undergo TURP [31]. Conversely, there have been several recent retrospective studies that have demonstrated improved symptom scores, quality of life, and post-void residual in men with DU treated with TURP or laser enucleation of the prostate. However, symptom improvement was less marked compared to previously published results in men with BOO in absence of DU [32, 33]. Additionally, the

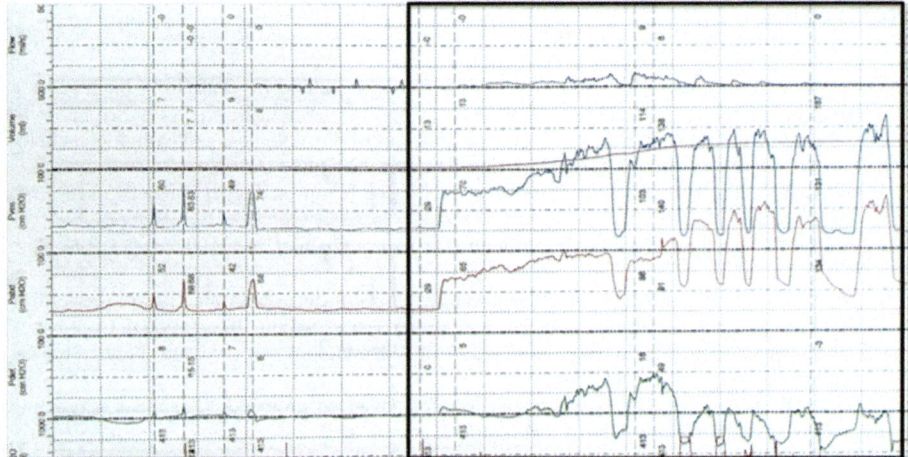

Fig. 7 Acontractile bladder with minimal flow due to repeated volitional increases in abdominal pressure (Valsalva voiding)

presence of concomitant detrusor overactivity and the presence of ultrastructural detrusor changes have been identified as predictors of poorer outcomes following surgical treatment for BOO [34–36].

In low-flow states, a valsalva maneuver is often used to increase the abdominal pressure and consequently the vesicle pressure in an attempt to overcome poor bladder emptying (Fig. 7). Patients with severe bladder outlet obstruction or detrusor underactivity sometimes rely on this added pressure to improve bladder emptying. Abdominal pressure is seen to rise in both of these conditions during voiding. Differentiation between outlet obstruction and detrusor activity is determined by identifying a high or low detrusor pressure, respectively, during the voiding phase as patients with outlet obstruction with a normal functioning bladder will maintain the ability to generate significant detrusor pressures.

Conclusion

Methodical evaluation of the pressure-flow phase of urodynamic studies provides valuable, objective evidence of obstructive voiding patterns. Additionally, valuable information about detrusor function is obtained which can aid in better categorizing patient voiding dysfunction. Urodynamic data obtained during the voiding phase can be applied to mathematical equations and nomograms to further characterize patients and help guide treatment planning.

References

1. Gleason DM, Lattimer JK. The pressure-flow study: a method for measuring bladder neck resistance. J Urol. 1962;87:844–52.
2. Schäfer W. Urethral resistance? Urodynamic concepts of physiological and pathological bladder outlet function during voiding. NeurourolUrodyn. 1985;4(3):161–201.
3. Conrad WA. Pressure–flow relationships in collapsible tubes. IEEE Trans Biomed Eng. 1969;16(4):284–95.
4. Griffiths DJ. Urethral elasticity and micturition hydrodynamics in females. Med Biol Eng. 1969;7(2):201–15.
5. Griffiths D, et al. Standardization of terminology of lower urinary tract function: pressure-flow studies of voiding, urethral resistance, and urethral obstruction. International Continence Society Subcommittee on Standardization of Terminology of Pressure-Flow Studies. NeurourolUrodyn. 1997;16(1):1–18.
6. Schäfer W. Principles and clinical application of advanced urodynamic analysis of voiding function. Urol Clin North Am. 1990;17(3):553–66.
7. Griffiths DJ. Hydrodynamics of male micturition. I. Theory of steady flow through elastic-walled tubes. Med Biol Eng. 1971;9(6):581–8.
8. Griffiths DJ. The mechanics of the urethra and of micturition. Br J Urol. 1973;45(5):497–507.
9. Nitti VW. Pressure flow urodynamic studies: the gold standard for diagnosing bladder outlet obstruction. Rev Urol. 2005;7 Suppl 6:S14–21.
10. Blaivas J. Multichannel urodynamic studies. Urology. 1984;23(5):421–38.
11. Abrams PH, Griffiths DJ. The assessment of prostatic obstruction from urodynamic measurements and from residual urine. Br J Urol. 1979;51(2):129–34.
12. Griffiths D. Basics of pressure-flow studies. World J Urol. 1995;13(1):30–3.
13. Lim CS, Abrams P. The Abrams-Griffiths nomogram. World J Urol. 1995;13(1):34–9.
14. Cox L, Jaffe WI. Urodynamics in male LUTS: when are they necessary and how do we use them? Urol Clin North Am. 2014;41(3):399–407.
15. Sekido N. Bladder contractility and urethral resistance relation: what does a pressure flow study tell us? Int J Urol. 2012;19(3):216–28.
16. Javle P, et al. Grading of benign prostatic obstruction can predict the outcome of transurethral prostatectomy. J Urol. 1998;160(5):1713–7.
17. Gotoh M, et al. Prognostic value of pressure-flow study in surgical treatment of benign prostatic obstruction. World J Urol. 1999;17(5):274–8.
18. Rodrigues P, et al. Urodynamic pressure flow studies can predict the clinical outcome after transurethral prostatic resection. J Urol. 2001;165(2):499–502.
19. Onyishi SE, Twiss CO. Pressure flow studies in men and women. Urol Clin North Am. 2014;41(3):453–67.
20. Scarpero H. Urodynamics in the evaluation of female LUTS: when are they helpful and how do we use them? Urol Clin North Am. 2014;41(3):429–38.
21. Carlson KV, Fiske J, Nitti VW. Value of routine evaluation of the voiding phase when performing urodynamic testing in women with lower urinary tract symptoms. J Urol. 2000;164(5):1614–8.
22. Monz B, et al. Patient characteristics associated with quality of life in European women seeking treatment for urinary incontinence: results from PURE. Eur Urol. 2007;51(4):1073–81. discussion 1081–2.
23. Irwin DE, et al. Population-based survey of urinary incontinence, overactive bladder, and other lower urinary tract symptoms in five countries: results of the EPIC study. Eur Urol. 2006;50(6):1306–14. discussion 1314–5.
24. Defreitas GA, et al. Refining diagnosis of anatomic female bladder outlet obstruction: comparison of pressure-flow study parameters in clinically obstructed women with those of normal controls. Urology. 2004;64(4):675–9. discussion 679–81.

25. Nitti VW, Tu LM, Gitlin J. Diagnosing bladder outlet obstruction in women. J Urol. 1999;161(5):1535–40.
26. Blaivas JG, Groutz A. Bladder outlet obstruction nomogram for women with lower urinary tract symptomatology. NeurourolUrodyn. 2000;19(5):553–64.
27. Groutz A, Blaivas JG. Bladder outlet obstruction in women: definition and characteristics. NeurourolUrodyn. 2000;19(3):213–20.
28. Osman NI, et al. Detrusor underactivity and the underactive bladder: a new clinical entity? A review of current terminology, definitions, epidemiology, aetiology, and diagnosis. Eur Urol. 2014;65(2):389–98.
29. Schäfer W. Analysis of bladder-outlet function with the linearized passive urethral resistance relation, linPURR, and a disease-specific approach for grading obstruction: from complex to simple. World J Urol. 1995;13(1):47–58.
30. Abrams P. Bladder outlet obstruction index, bladder contractility index and bladder voiding efficiency: three simple indices to define bladder voiding function. BJU Int. 1999;84(1):14–5.
31. Thomas AW, et al. The natural history of lower urinary tract dysfunction in men: the influence of detrusor underactivity on the outcome after transurethral resection of the prostate with a minimum 10-year urodynamic follow-up. BJU Int. 2004;93(6):745–50.
32. Mitchell CR, et al. Efficacy of holmium laser enucleation of the prostat in patients with non-neurogenic impaired bladder: results of a prospective trial. Urology. 2014;83(2):428–32.
33. Han DH, et al. The efficacy of transurethral resection of the prostate in the patients with weak bladder contractility index. Urology. 2008;71(4):657–61.
34. Blatt AH, et al. Transurethral prostate resection in patients with hypocontractile detrusor–what is the predictive value of ultrastructural detrusor changes? J Urol. 2012;188(6):2294–9.
35. Seki N, et al. Predictives regarding outcome after transurethral resection for prostatic adenoma associated with detrusor underactivity. URL. 2006;67(2):306–10.
36. Tanaka Y, et al. Is the short-term outcome of transurethral resection of the prostate affected by preoperative degree of bladder outlet obstruction, status of detrusor contractility or detrusor overactivity? Int J Urol. 2006;13(11):1398–404.

The EMG

Kristy M. Borawski

History of Electromyography (EMG)

In the 1950, DISA A/S (Copenhagen, Denmark) introduced model 13A67, a 3-channel system for EMG recordings. The first fiber-optic recorder with instant capture and visualization of EMG recordings was introduced in 1966. This was then followed by digital systems, microprocessor controlled EMG systems and finally, the PC-based EMG systems emerged after 1993 [1].

Clinical Indications

Sphincter electromyography is an indirect measure of pelvic floor and urethral muscle sphincter activity. This is a measurement of the depolarization of the sphincter muscle membrane [2, 3]. This depolarization, originally described by DuBois, and its electrical current, first measured by von Helmoltz in 1850, pioneered modern EMG tracings [4].

Measurement of pelvic floor muscle function is an integral component of a urodynamics study especially in light of neurologic, gynecologic or trauma related factors that may impair the lower urinary tract function. Questions that can be answered include information on outlet contraction and relaxation in relation to the timing of other components of the urodynamics study [2]. **In the most recent American Urological Association/Society of Urodynamics and Female Urology guidelines on adult urodynamics, EMG was recommend in combination with a cystometrogram with or without a pressure flow study in patients with relevant**

K.M. Borawski, M.D. (✉)
Department of Urology, University of North Carolina—Chapel Hill,
2113 Physicians Office Building, Campus Box 7235, Chapel Hill, NC 27599, USA
e-mail: kristy_borawski@med.unc.edu

neurologic disease at risk for neurogenic bladder or in patients with other neurologic disease and elevated PVR or urinary symptoms [5]. It may also aid in the evaluation of neurologically intact individuals with obstructive pressure flow studies in the absence of an anatomical obstruction [6].

Selecting the Appropriate EMG Measurement Tool

Measuring the electrical potential variations in muscles can be done with respect to an unchanging reference value (monopolar) or as the potential difference between two points (bipolar) [7]. **Three main kinds of electrodes for EMG measurement are available for use; needle, surface and wire electrodes.** Concentric needle electrodes (CNE) consist of a hollow steel needle within which is a fine wire insulated except at its tip. The potential difference between the outer and inner core is measured while the patient is grounded with a separate surface electrode [8]. Concentric needles are placed into the peri-urethral muscle near the urethral muscle in women (placed just lateral to the urethral meatus and advanced parallel for 1–2 cm) and the bulbocavernosus muscle in men. Placement can be confirmed by an audio monitor which will demonstrate a popping noise that increases if the patient is asked to contract their pelvic muscles [4]. **Needle electrodes can isolate electrical activity from specific muscle fibers within a 0.5 mm radius of the tip and remain the standard for measuring neuromuscular activity** [9, 10]. Difficulties with correct needle placement, patient discomfort and limitation of patient mobility during urodynamic testing to avoid dislodging the needles all limit the usefulness of CNE in the clinical setting [10]. However, needles also allow for oscilloscope monitoring allowing for analysis of individual action potentials.

An alternative to CNEs, are thin steel, platinum or copper wires that are inserted into the pelvic floor using 25-gauge needles). The needle is then withdrawn leaving the wire, with a small hook, within the pelvic floor musculature. Similarly to CNEs, wires are placed into the periurethral muscle of the female patient or the bulbocavernosus muscle in the male patient and the use of audio monitor is recommended while placing the wires. **Unlike with CNEs, wires cannot be manipulated once placed and if they are placed incorrectly or become dislodged, they must be removed and replaced. As with CNEs, technical placement errors, patient discomfort and limitation of patient movement are limiting factors in utilizing wires for EMG evaluation** [4, 11].

Barrett first described the use of disposable infant surface electrodes as an indirect indicator of external urethral sphincter function [10, 12]. The use of the external anal sphincter has been reported to be a reliable means of evaluating the external urethral sphincter activity in patients who have no evidence for pelvic trauma or diffuse demyelinating disease [13–15]. Several surface electrodes are available for use; however, smaller (infant) patches are preferred because they can be placed closer to the anal verge. Polymer based backings are preferable to gel foam backings as the latter is an effective insulator and may interfere with EMG signals.

Silver or silver-chloride surface EMGs are good conductors and may help minimize motion artifact produced by skin potentials [16, 17]. Surface EMGs are available as patches with shielded cables or unshielded wires with reusable snaps. The former are preferable as they avoid potential artifact when exposed to urinary flow or noise. Two active plates should be placed as close to the anal verge possible, however, if using unshielded patches, use care to avoid contact between the wire snaps. A grounding electrode is placed on a near muscular area such as the tendon of the thigh serving as a grounding electrode. Prior to placement, the skin should be prepped. Although rubbing the skin with medical abrasive paste results in the best site preparation, it is often not tolerated by the patient [4, 17]. Using a perineal cleaner or soap with gauze is preferred over alcohol as alcohol based cleaners can increase impedance in EMG signals. Surface EMG electrode placement is confirmed by asking the patient to contract the pelvic floor muscles and cough. EMG signal should increase during these events [4].

Several studies have compared concentric needle EMG electrode to surface electrodes. One of the main drawbacks to the use of surface EMG electrodes which rely on peri-anal muscle signals is the validity of using this muscle as a surrogate for urethral sphincter activity. Several studies have demonstrated separate innervation of the levator ani and urethral sphincter. This suggests that perineal measurements of levator ani will not accurately reflect urethral sphincter activity [10, 15, 18]. Barrett examined the use of surface EMG electrodes in two separate studies and demonstrated that surface EMG electrodes showed grossly similar findings to peri-anal wire electrodes and that adequately detected perineal relaxation when attempting to diagnose neurological voiding dysfunction [10, 19]. However, several studies directly comparing concentric needle to surface EMG electrodes dispute the validity and reliability of surface EMG electrodes. The compound muscle action potentials are smaller with the use of surface EMG electrodes and as such, the signal needs larger amplification. This can result in poorer signal to noise ratio. Similarly, multiple studies have shown a functional dissociation between the separate branches of the pudendal nerve innervating the levator ani and urethral sphincter. Thus, we may not be able to rely on EMG signals obtained from the external anal sphincter as a true representation of urethral sphincter activity [14, 15, 20–22]. Therefore, the use of concentric needle EMG electrodes may provide for the most accurate assessment of external urethral sphincter activity, although it does come at a potential cost of patient discomfort and easy dislodgement of the needle with patient movement during the test.

Sources of Potential Artifact in EMG Tracings

Electromyography is susceptible to potential artifacts created by electrical currents that are not generated from the targeted motor units. The environment during EMG testing is a rich source of potential artifacts. Electrical noise that may affect an EMG signal can be divided into several categories: Inherent noise,

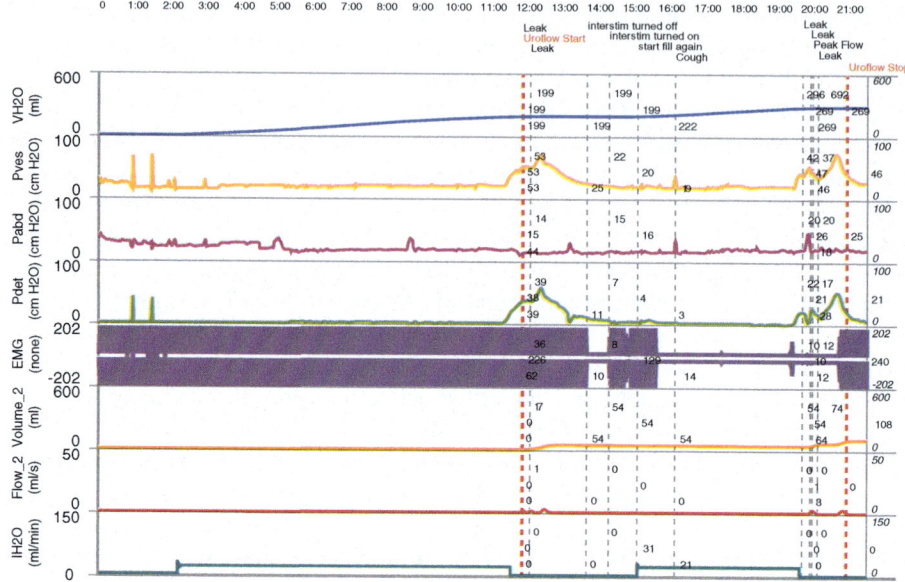

Fig. 1 Effects of sacral neuromodulation (SNM) on EMG tracing

ambient noise and motion artifact. Inherent noise is the noise that all electronic equipment generates and cannot be altered. If it is interfering with the EMG test (the clinician can attach a surface EMG electrode to their hand and engage each potential source), it should be turned off, removed or modified to prevent significant artifact on the EMG testing. Common sources for electrical noise include 60 Hz signals from room lighting, fluoroscopic generators, electrosurgical units and microwave ovens. Ambient noise is caused by electromagnetic radiation. Motion artifact is usually caused by movement of the electrode interface or the electrode cables [4, 13, 23]. **Another modern source of artifact is a sacral neuromodulation device. While on, it will interfere with the EMG signal but the signal reverts to normal when the device is turned off** (Fig. 1).

Physiologic artifact may also interfere with EMG tracings. The most common cause of artifact is the EMG signal generated from the heart. It will take on the pattern of the patients pulse rate. Significant lower extremity spasms as can be seen in patients with neurologic insults can also result in EMG artifact. While these potential sources of artifact can be identified, they usually cannot be removed from the EMG study.

The most common source of artifact is technical factors. These include improper electrode placement and/or improper grounding. This potential source of error can be minimized by proper insertion technique either employing the use of an audio monitor when feasible or by testing placement by having the patient cough or actively recruit pelvic musculature. The clinician should have a low threshold for re-evaluating electrode placement throughout the urodynamic study and replacing and/or repositioning the electrodes as necessary. Another source of technical artifact is voiding across surface EMG electrodes resulting in an increase in EMG signal. Taping of the lead wires in unshielded patches or using shielded patches may help to decrease this potential source of error [4].

Normal EMG Behavior During Voiding

Electromyography should be recorded throughout the urodynamics test including bladder filling, provocative maneuvers and during voiding. The patient without neurological sequalae should be able to show an increase in EMG tracing during a cough or valsalva maneuver (Fig. 2). Although common, not all patients will be able to recruit pelvic floor musculature (and hence increase EMG signal) when asked to perform a volitional Kegels exercise. In fact, several studies have shown that 30–70 % of patients may not be able to recruit their pelvic floor musculature when volitionally asked [24, 25].

During bladder filling, the EMG signal should stay relatively quiet and consistent. You may note a slight increase in resting EMG tone throughout bladder filling, a process called recruitment or the guarding reflex [26]. This reflex may be heightened in spinal cord injured patients (Fig. 3).

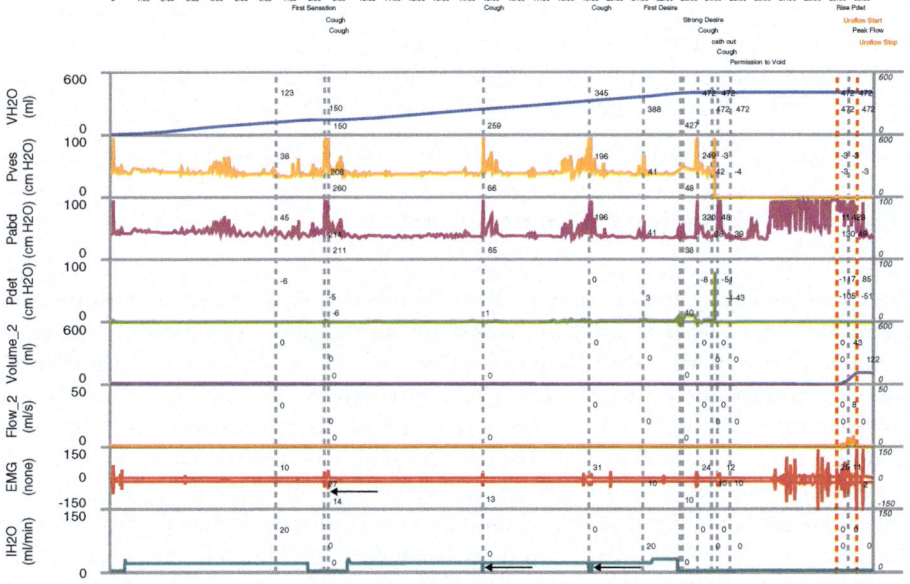

Fig. 2 EMG response to cough. Note increase in EMG signal with cough/valsalva (*arrows*)

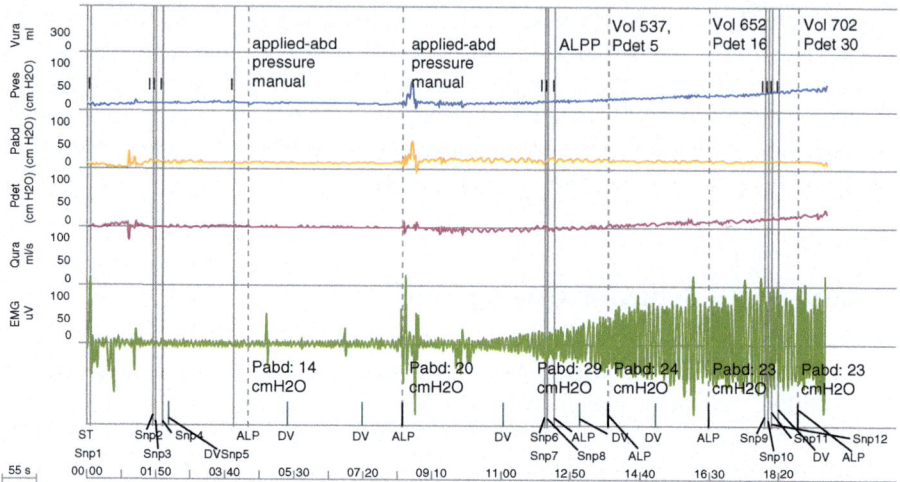

Fig. 3 Exaggerated recruitment (guarding reflex) during bladder filling in a spinal cord injured patient

During normal micturition, EMG activity disappears completely for a few seconds before a detrusor contraction starts. This is coordinated in response to neuromodulation by the pontine micturition center. The EMG signal then resumes once the bladder is empty [26]. However, in a secondary analysis of urodynamic and EMG data from the SISTEr trial, quantitative and qualitative EMG signals during urine flow were usually greater than during fill. There did not seem to be a correlation to post operative voiding dysfunction and higher preoperative EMG activity. The authors noted that in this group of women, perineal surface patch EMG did not measure the expected pelvic floor and urethral sphincter relaxation during voiding [27].

Abnormal Behavior During Voiding

Electromyography testing may be most helpful in those patients with neurogenic disorders as it is useful to assist in the diagnosis of detrusor external sphincter dyssynergia that is characterized by an involuntary contraction of the external sphincter during detrusor contraction. This is characterized by an increase in EMG signal during the micturition phase associated with a detrusor contraction. It is commonly seen in suprasacral spinal cord lesions such as spinal cord injury, multiple sclerosis, thoracic myelomeningocele, transverse myelitis, and other lesions that interfere with neuromodulation from the pontine micturition center. Detrusor sphincter dyssynergia, if not managed appropriately, may have negative effects of both the upper and lower urinary tract, the extent of which is beyond the scope of this chapter.

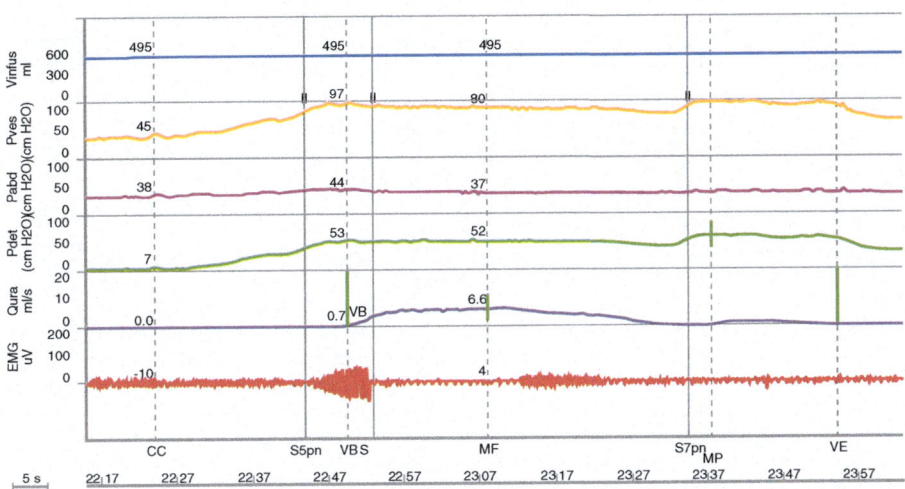

Fig. 4 Type 1 detrusor sphincter dyssynergia (note slight volitional increase towards latter part of the void)

Blaivis described three types of detrusor sphincter dyssynergia (DSD) Type 1 DSD (Fig. 4), demonstrated in 30 % of his study population, was characterized by a crescendo increase in EMG activity that reached a maximum at the peak of the detrusor contraction. Type 2 DSD (Fig. 5) consisted of clonic sphincter contractions interspersed throughout the detrusor contraction and type 3 DSD (Fig. 6) (55 % of his study population) was characterized by a sustained sphincter contraction that coincided with the detrusor contraction. No correlation was noted to spinal cord injury level (all were suprasacral) and pattern of DSD.

It is important to consider that some volitional behaviors such as recruitment of pelvic floor due to pain or discomfort (Fig. 7), an increase in EMG signal in response to valsalva/Crede voiding or any other source of artifact (fluid on patch, etc.) may mimic detrusor sphincter dyssynergia. Careful attention to these factors during the procedure is important to prevent misinterpretation of the results. It is this authors practice to repeat the test using fluoroscopy (see chapter "The Use of Fluoroscopy" for more details), if not already in use, if an unexpected increase in EMG signal was noted without any identifiable artifact. Several studies have demonstrated that fluoroscopic images can significant assist in the diagnosis of detrusor sphincter dyssynergia in the setting of a potentially unreliable surface patch EMG electrode [22].

The confirmed, unexpected finding of an increase in EMG signal during micturition should prompt a neurologic evaluation to look for an underlying source such as multiple sclerosis. **If no neurologic source is found in the presence of increased sphincter activity with voiding, the diagnosis of dysfunctional voiding or pelvic floor dyssynergia is applied** [28]. **Dysfunctional voiding is defined as 'intermittent and/or fluctuating flow rate due to involuntary intermittent contractions of the peri-urethral striated muscle during voiding in neurologically normal individuals'** [29]. Fowlers syndrome is a subgroup of women with

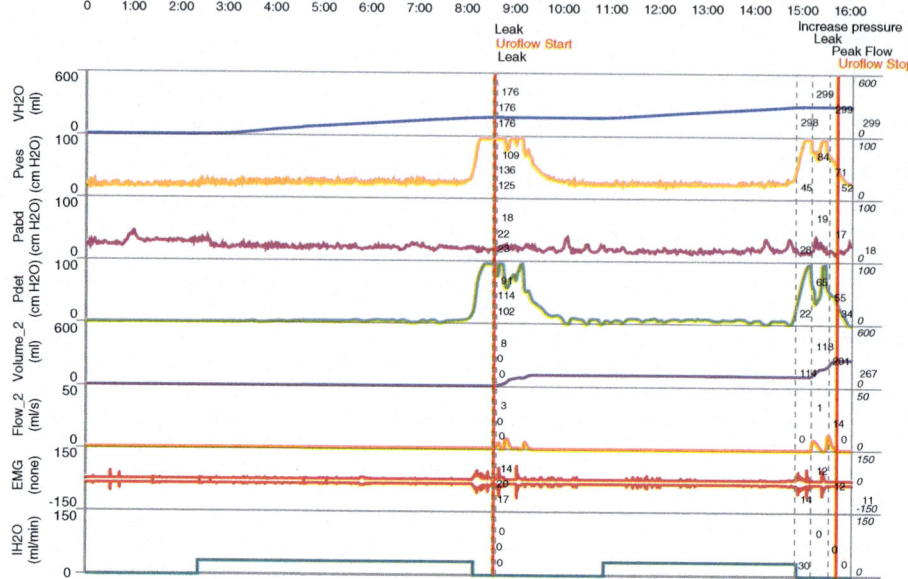

Fig. 5 Type 2 detrusor sphincter dyssynergia

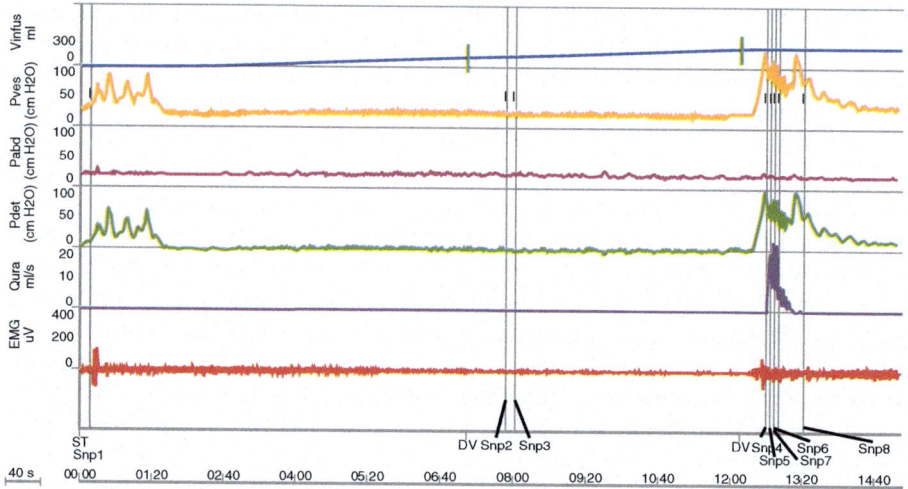

Fig. 6 Type 3 detrusor sphincter dyssynergia

dysfunctional voiding that present with urinary retention and often endocrine problems resembling Stein-Leventhal syndrome. These women may show characteristic non-relaxing EMG during voiding or an increase in EMG signal during micturition. There is no identifiable neurologic lesion that can account for the increase in EMG signal [30].

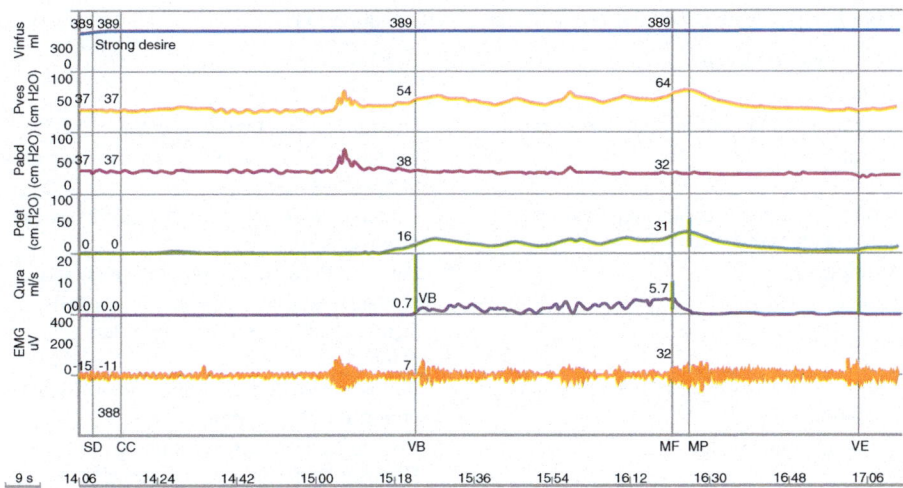

Fig. 7 Volitional increase in EMG signal during voiding. This does not represent type 2 DSD. This was identified by querying the patient during the study

With sacral or infra-sacral denervation injuries such as radial pelvic surgery or sacral myelomeningocele, the urethra may have a fixed, non-relaxing tone. No significant change will be noted on EMG signal during the filling or micturition phases of the urodynamic study.

Electromyography is an important component in the urodynamic study of patients with Parkinson's disease or Multiple System Atrophy (MSA, Shy-Drager Syndrome). Sphincter bradykinesia, defined as an involuntary increase in EMG signal that persists through at least the initial part of the expulsive phase of the bladder [31]. This is a fairly common finding in Parkinson's disease. The prevalence of detrusor sphincter dyssynergia is low (0–3 %) in Parkinson's patients [32]. In MSA, due to neuronal loss in the sacral Onuf's nucleus, there is a denervation injury of the external urethral sphincter. This results in prolonged motor unit potential (MUP) duration. Palace et al., classified a neurogenic MUP as one that has >20 % of MUP duration more than 10 ms (normal is 3–8 ms) or an average MUP duration of >10 ms [33].

Table 1 reviews several neurologic conditions and their potential EMG findings.

Conclusion

Electromyography can aid in the diagnosis of various causes of voiding dysfunction, both neurogenic and non-neurogenic. However, it is a technically challenging, often non-specific component of requires a clear understanding of the patient's history.

Table 1 Neurologic conditions and anticipated EMG findings [34]

Neurologic condition	EMG findings
Suprapontine lesion	Coordinated EMG
Suprasacral, sub-pontine spinal cord lesion	Destrusor sphincter dyssynergia
Sacral lesion	Potential dennervation, either no change or prolonged MUP
Infrasacral lesion (i.e. radical pelvic surgery, abdominoperineal resection)	Potential dennervation, either no change or prolonged MUP
Multiple sclerosis	Potential for detrusor sphincter dyssynergia
Parkinson's disease	Sphincter bradykinesia (more common) Detrusor sphincter dyssynergia (less common)
Multiple System Atrophy (MSA) Shy-Drager Syndrome	Prolonged MUP (>20 % more than 10 ms or average MUP>10 ms)
Traumatic brain injury	Coordinated sphincter (common) Detrusor sphincter dyssynergia (if brain stem injury)
Cerebral palsy	Coordinated sphincter (common)
Dementia	Coordinated sphincter
Spinal dysraphism	Detrusor sphincter dyssynergia (30–40 %)

EMG data should be interpreted in the context of the patient's history, physical examination findings, fluoroscopic, cystometric and uroflowmetry data to obtain the most useful information [5].

References

1. Ladengaard J. Sorty of eletromyography equipment. Muscle Nerve Supp. 2002;11:S128–33.
2. Lenherr SM, Clemons JC. Urodynamics. Urol Clin N Am. 2013;40(4):545–57.
3. Mayo ME. Value of sphincter electromyography in urodynamics. J Urol. 1979;122(3):357–60.
4. Gray M. Traces: making sense of urodynamics testing – Part 3. Electromyeography of the pelvic floor muscles. Urol Nurs. 2011;31(3):31–8.
5. Winters JC, Dmochowski RR, Goldman HB, Anthony Herndon CD, Kobashi KC, Kraus SR, Lemack GE, Nitti VN, Rovner ES, Wein AJ. Urodynamnic studies in adults: AUA/SUFU guideline. J Urol. 2012;188:2462–72.
6. Brucker BM, Fong E, Shah S, Kelly C, Rosenblum N, Nitti V. Urodynamics differences between dysfunctional voiding and primary bladder neck obstruction in women. Urology. 2012;80(1):55–60.
7. Rowant D, James ED, Kramer AWJL, Sterling AM, Suhel PF. International Continence Society working party on urodynamic equipment. J Med Eng Technol. 1987;11:57–64.
8. Blavias JG. Sphincter electromyopgraphy. Neurol Urodyn. 1983;2:269–88.
9. Mahajan ST, Fitzgerald MP, Kenton K, Shott S, Brubaker L. Concentric needle electrodes are superior to perineal surface-patch electrodes for electromyographic documentation of urethral sphincter relaxation during voiding. BJU Int. 2006;97:117–20.
10. Bradley CS, Smith KE, Kreder KJ. Urodynamic evaluation of the bladder and pelvic floor. Gastroenterol Clin N Am. 2008;37:539–52.

11. Siroky MB. Electromyography of the perineal floor. Urol Clin N Am. 1996;23:299–307.
12. Barrett DM. Disposable (infant) surface electrocardiogram electrodes in urodynamics: a simultaneous comparative studies of electrodes. J Urol. 1980;125:538–41.
13. O'Donnell P, Beck C, Doyle R, Eubanks C. Surface electrodes in perineal electromyography. Urology. 1998;32(4):375–9.
14. Perkash I. Urodynamic evaluation: periurethral striated EMG versus perianal striated EMG. Paraplegia. 1980;18:275.
15. Vereecken RL, Verduyn H. The electrical activity of the paraurethral and perineal muscles in normal and pathological conditions. Br J Urol. 1970;42:457.
16. Webster JG. Reducing motion artifact and interference in biopotential recordings. IEE Trans BioMed Eng. 1984;31:823–6.
17. Bolek JE. Electrical concepts in the surface electromyographic signal. App Psychophysiol Biofeedback. 2010;35:171–5.
18. Barber MD, Bremer RE, Thor KB, Dolber PC, Kuehl TJ, Coates KW. Inneraction of the female levator ani muscles. Am J Obstet Gynecol. 2002;187:64–71.
19. Barrett DM, Wein AJ. Flow evaluation and simultaneous external sphincter electromyography in clinical urodynamics. J Urol. 1981;125:538–41.
20. Brostrom S, Jennum P, Lose G. Motor evoked potentials from the striated urethral sphincter: a comparison of concentric needle and surface electrodes. Neurol Urodyn. 2003;22:123–9.
21. Blavas JG, Labib KL, Bauer SB, Retik AB. A new approach to electromyography of the external urethral sphincter. J Urol. 1977;117:773–7.
22. Be EJ, Patel CY, Tharian B, Westney OK, Grawe PE, Hairston JC. Diagnostic discordance of electromyography (EMG) versus voiding cystourethrogram (VCUG) for detrusor-external sphincter dyssynergy (DESD). Neuourol Urodyn. 2005;24(7):616–21.
23. Raez MBI, Hussain MS, Mohd-Yasin F. Techniques of EMG signal analysis, detection, processing, classification and applications. Biol Proced Online. 2006;8:11–35.
24. Berghmans LCM, Freferiks CMA, de Bie RA, Weil EHJ, Smeets LWH, Van Waalwijk ESC, Janknegt RA. Efficacy of biofeedback, when included with pelvic floor muscle exercise treatment for genuine stress incontinence. Neuourol Urodyn. 1996;15:37–52.
25. Bump RC, Hurt WG, Fantl JA, Wyman JF. Assessment of Kegel pelvic muscle exercise performance after brief verbal instruction. Am J Obstet Gynecol. 1991;165(2):322–9.
26. Mahfouz W, Al Afraa T, Campeau L, Corcos J. Normal urodynamic parameters in women. Int Urogynecol J. 2012;23:269–77.
27. Kriby AC, Nager CW, Litman HL, FitzGerald MP, Kraus S, Norton P, Sirls L, Rickey L, Wilson T, Dandreo KJ, Shepherd J, Zimmern P. Perineal surface electromyography does not typically demonstrate the expected relaxation during normal voiding. Neuourol Urodyn. 2011; 30:1591–6.
28. Blaivas JG, Sinha HP, Zayed AA, Labib KB. Detrusor-external sphincter dyssynergia: a detailed electromyographic study. J Urol. 1981;125(4):545–9.
29. Abrams P, Cardozo L, Fall M, Griffiths D, Rosier P, Ulmsten U, van Kerrebroeck P, Victor A, Wein A, Standardisation Sub-committee of the International Continence Society. The standardisation of terminology of lower urinary tract function: report from the Standardisation Subcommittee of the International Continence Society. Neurourol Urodyn. 2002;21(2):167–78.
30. Fowler CJ, Christmas T, Chapple CR, Fitzmaurice H, Kirby RS, Jacobs HS. Abnormal electromyographic activity of the urethral sphincter, voiding dysfunction and polycystic ovaries: a new syndrome? BMJ. 1988;297:1436–8.
31. Pavlakis AJ, Siroky MB, Goldstein I. Neurourologic findings in Parkinson's disease. J Urol. 1983;129:80.
32. Lee D, Dillon B, Lemack GE. LUTS in the patient with Parkinson's disease. AUA Update Ser. 2012; 31(Lesson 38):377–84.
33. Palace J, Chandiramani VA, Fowler CJ. Value of sphincter electromyography in the diagnosis of multiple system atrophy. Muscle Neuro. 1997;20:1296–403.
34. Wein AJ. Pathophysiology and classification of lower urinary tract dysfunction. In: Wein AJ, Kavoussi LR, Novick AC, Partin AW, Peters CA, editors. Campbell-Walsh urology. Philadelphia, PA: Saunders; 2012. p. 1834–46.

The Use of Fluoroscopy

Tom Feng and Karyn S. Eilber

Introduction

One of the main goals of urodynamics is to provide the clinician with information as to the pathophysiology of a patient's symptoms. A simple urodynamics study includes only a single-channel cystometrogram (CMG) and is used to assess bladder pressure alone. Complex, or multi-channel, urodynamic studies combine CMG with flow and intraabdominal pressure. Electromyography (EMG) and the urethral pressure profile are also often included in multi-channel urodynamic studies. For both simple and complex urodynamics, the fluid medium is typically sterile water or saline.

Addition of lower urinary tract imaging to complex urodynamics, usually fluoroscopy, is referred to as avideourodynamic study (VUDS).A videourodynamic study consists of the simultaneous measurement of multi-channel urodynamic parameters with imaging of the lower urinary tract. It provides precise evaluation of both lower urinary tract anatomy and function. The fluid medium for VUDS is radiographic contrast. The additional data provided by real time radiographic imaging can be essential in making accurate diagnoses.

Universally accepted criteria regarding patient selection for complex urodynamics or videourodynamic studies do not exist and are mainly based on expert opinion. However, the 2012 American urologic Association guidelines on urodynamics clearly state that urodynamics are indicated when 1) an accurate diagnosis cannot

---

T. Feng, M.D.
Department of Surgery, Division of Urology, Cedars-Sinai Medical Center,
8635 W. 3rd St., Suite 1070, Los Angeles, CA 90048, USA
e-mail: tom.feng@cshs.org

K.S. Eilber, M.D. (✉)
Department of Surgery, Division of Urology, Cedars-Sinai Medical Center,
99 N. La Cienega Boulevard, Suite 307, Beverly Hills, CA 90211, USA
e-mail: karyn.eilber@cshs.org

© Springer International Publishing Switzerland 2016
A.C. Peterson, M.O. Fraser (eds.), *Practical Urodynamics for the Clinician*,
DOI 10.1007/978-3-319-20834-3_8

be made by history, physical, and preliminary testing and invasive and/or irreversible treatment is being considered, 2) empiric or definitive treatment has failed, 3) a patient's lower urinary tract dysfunction has the potential to cause upper tract deterioration and 4) when considering invasive, potentially morbid and nonreversible interventions [1, 2].

Fluoroscopic Imaging of the Lower Urinary Tract

Dynamic imaging of the lower urinary tract dates as far back as the 1960s in the form of cineradiography [3, 4]. Although this type of imaging provided desired information, the procedure had to be performed in a radiology department and was associated with relatively high rates of radiation exposure. Fluoroscopy for the lower urinary tract gained favor as more portable devices were introduced and allowed for radiographic studies to be performed in the ambulatory setting.

Videourodynamic tests are still often performed in a radiology department due to cost and personnel, but modern-day fluoroscopy units are compact and mobile and thus ideal for office use. Commercial software is available that correlates fluoroscopic images with the corresponding urodynamic parameters such that reports have the image alongside the pressure tracing.

Requirements for Fluoroscopy Use

The requirements for use of fluoroscopy have regional variations, but typical requirements include practitioner licensing, machine registration, and radiation shielding of the examination room and personnel. The following information is based on the authors' local and state requirements.

Practitioner Licensing

Licensing for use of fluoroscopy varies by state. In the authors' state, a Radiology Supervisor and Operator Certificate or a Fluoroscopy Supervisor and Operator Permit are required for any health care personnel who directly operate or supervise the operation of fluoroscopy equipment, position the patient during fluoroscopy, or determine radiation exposure to a patient during fluoroscopy procedures [5].

Competence in the areas of radiation safety and image acquisition is documented by receipt of appropriate licensure. In order to obtain such credentials, the physician must demonstrate competency in radiation protection and in the safe use of fluoroscopy either through an examination process or continuing medical education credits. Personnel who do not possess appropriate licensure to operate fluoroscopic equipment should not use the machine in any capacity. Most states require that a current copy of the licensure be posted.

Facility Requirements

Similar to practitioner licensing, each state has different requirements as to the necessity of lead shielding in the walls that house the fluoroscopy equipment [6]. Doors must also be closed during fluoroscopy to act as a radiation barrier. **Although state requirements may vary, a common rule is that if the fluoroscopy unit will be routinely used in one location then shielding must be provided in the form of 1.5 mm of lead or equivalent shielding material. If shielding is required, aradiationphysicist is necessary to evaluate the site and submit a shielding design to your local regulatory agency.**

Machine Requirements

The U.S. Food and Drug Administration (FDA) regulates the manufacturers of all x-ray imaging devices through requirements for personnel qualification, quality assurance, and facility accreditation [7]. Owners of the fluoroscopic equipment must register with the state in accordance of its provisions. In general, safety inspections occur annually and are administered by local regulatory agencies.

Radiation Safety

An important principlewhenperforming any radiologic procedure is for the study to be performed with the highest quality to produce the desired image while minimizing the amount of radiation exposure. The concept of ALARA (As Low As Reasonably Achievable) implies that, whenever possible, radiation exposure should be minimized [8].

Documenting the amount of radiation exposure during fluoroscopic procedures is mandatory. All personnel who perform fluoroscopy must wear a radiation monitoring device such as a film badge. If the machine operator does not stand behind a protective barrier, then a lead apron must be worn with a minimum of 0.25 mm of lead equivalent. When procedures such as a retrograde urethrogram are frequently performed, consideration should be given to addition of protective gloves or eyewear.

Personnel who are likely to receive one-tenth of the annual maximum permissible levels from exposure to x-rays are provided a collar badge to be worn in front of the apron. It is likely that exposures will vary significantly between institutions and the private practice setting. Nevertheless, monitoring radiation dose allows comparison among users for quality improvement and to determine the adequacy of shielding and other protective measures.

The term collimation refers to limitation of the x-ray beam to the area of clinical interest. In doing so, this markedly reduces radiation exposure to the patient. Lack of collimation is one of the largest contributors to unnecessary patient radiation exposure. Similarly, the majority of fluoroscopy units are controlled by a "dead man" type exposure switch. With this switch the x-ray beam is active only when the operator is pressing the activation button and allows the operator to stand well away from the machine. Appropriate collimation and limitation of exposure time can keep patient radiation exposure to a minimum.

Factors such as kilovoltage (kVp) and milliampere-seconds (mAs) are usually preset in fluoroscopy machines to minimize the amount of radiation exposure. However, these values can be manipulated as with standard x-ray machines in appropriate circumstances in order to account for variations in patient body habitus. Table 1 shows the average radiation exposure of a fluoroscopic study during videourodynamics as compared to common imaging studies in urology [9, 10].

Advantages of Fluoroscopy

Multi-channel urodynamics without fluoroscopy provide a great deal of functional information, but there are several clinical scenarios for which fluoroscopy are of great value.

Anatomy

A videourodynamicsstudyis essential when anatomic information is needed to corroborate functional (urodynamic) observations. Fluoroscopic images for VUDS are typically obtained with the patient positioned for an anterior-posterior (AP) or lateral image. Positioning is mainly determined by clinical information that is desired, but patient body habitus and mobility limitations also influence positioning.

Table 1 Radiation exposure of commonly performed X-rays

Radiographic study	Typical radiation dose in millisieverts (mSv)
Chest X-ray	0.02–0.04
KUB	0.08
Fluoroscopy during VUDS	0.34
CT abdomen/pelvis	10–30
CT urogram	40

The Use of Fluoroscopy

Images necessary to diagnose incontinence, vesicoureteral reflux, and bladder outlet obstruction can usually be obtained with the AP position; however, accurate imaging of urethral abnormalities such as stricture disease is best performed in the lateral position as this affords the best visualization of the urethra.

Imaging Sequence

An initial *scout* film should be obtained. The main purpose of the scout film is for confirmation of desired patient position. Bony abnormalities are another finding that can be noted prior to initiation of the study. Attention should be paid to the spine when assessing patients with known or suspected neurogenic bladder. Surgical clips or other implants can provide information about prior procedures. Periodically a patient will have had other recent imaging with radiographic contrast. The baseline appearance of this must be noted to prevent misinterpretation of the VUDS findings.

After the bladder is partially filled with radiographic contrast, a *resting* image is obtained. This image provides additional useful information such as bladder shape and outline, bladder position at rest, bladder neck at rest, and abnormalities such as bladder diverticula (Fig. 1). The bladder outline is often irregular at volumes less than 200 mL because of external compression from adjacent bowel and pelvic organs [11]. If an abnormal finding is suspected to be due to external compression,

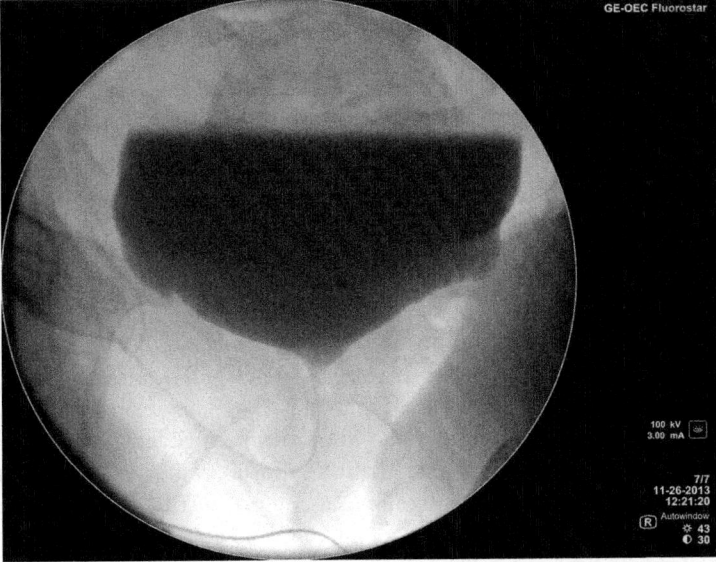

Fig. 1 Resting image of a woman with stress urinary incontinence. The bladder neck is open, and the bladder outline is irregular due to the bladder being only partially filled

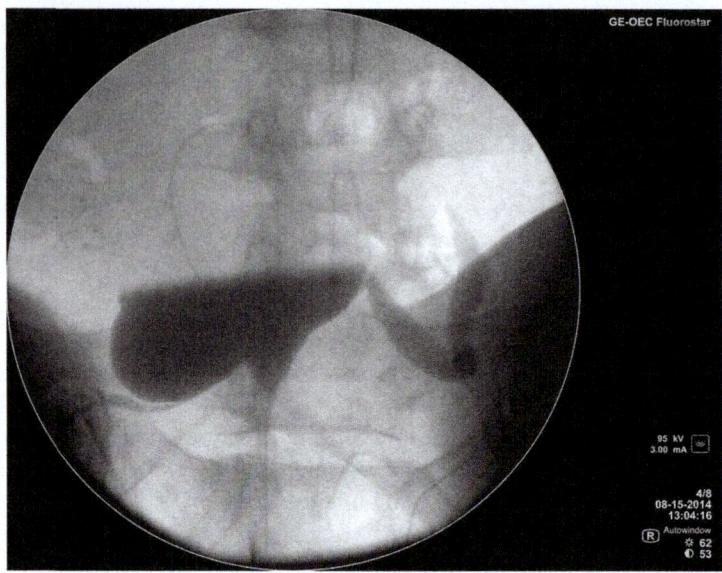

Fig. 2. Valsalva image of a woman with severe stress incontinence and declining renal function status post renal transplant. The bladder neck is totally incompetent, and there is reflux into the transplant kidney in the right pelvis and into the left native kidney

a repeat resting image should be obtained when the bladder has been filled with more contrast.

Once the resting image is acquired, a *strain (Valsalva)* or *cough* image is obtained. During straining, bladder neck competence and any associated incontinence (abdominal leak point pressure), degree of bladder descent (cystocele), and presence of vesicoureteral reflux can be assessed (Figs. 1 and 2).

When the bladder is filled to capacity, a*voiding cystourethrogram* **(VCUG)is performed.This portion of the VUDS is key when evaluating a patient for obstruction or when there is concern for high-pressure voiding causing reflux.** During this phase appropriate bladder neck and external sphincter relaxation and the urethral outline are observed. The presence of vesicoureteral reflux is again assessed. If stricture disease or other urethral pathology is suspected, the VCUG is best performed with the patient positioned such that a lateral image is obtained (Fig. 3a). If the VCUG is performed in the sitting position, a radiolucent chair is necessary. Female patients generally find it easier to void in a seated position, but if a woman is expected to void while standing then a funnel device is necessary.

Finally, a *post-void image* is obtained to determine bladder emptying (Fig. 3b). This image may be omitted to reduce radiation exposure if the post-void residual can be accurately determined based on volume of contrast instilled and volume voided or when the post-void residual is not a concern. The post-void image can also be useful to determine how much fluid is retained in a diverticulum after voiding.

Figure 4 shows the imagingsequence for VUDS.

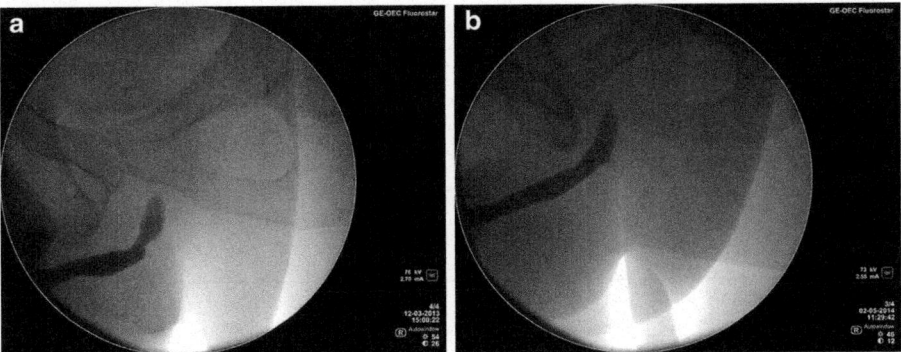

Fig. 3 (**a**) Lateral voiding film of a man with a urethral stricture. (**b**) The patient's postoperative voiding film

Incontinence

Patients with symptoms of mild stress incontinence that is not demonstrated by physical examination can have their diagnosis confirmed with a VUDS. **Even the smallest amount of incontinence can be detected with fluoroscopy.** On the contrary, the diagnosis of stress incontinence must be questioned when a patient's resting and straining images fail to demonstrate an open bladder neck. Studies have shown that presence of an open bladder neck correlates strongly with the presence of stress urinary incontinence [12]. In this study, none of the continent patients had an open bladder neck during a VUDS implying that a closed bladder neck should raise the suspicion that the patient has a diagnosis other than stress urinary incontinence.

In addition to providing information regarding the presence of incontinence, fluoroscopy also provides information as to the severity of incontinence. With a VUDS the amount of incontinence can be visually quantified and correlated with abdominal leak point pressure. This becomes relevant when a patient is presented with treatment options. A patient with incontinence of only a few drops of urine at a very high Valsalva leak point pressure (VLPP)may be an appropriate candidate for a bulking agent. On the other hand, a patient with a completely incompetent bladder neck who leaks with a minimal increase in abdominal pressure needs to consider closure of the bladder neck.

With the use of VUDS, the VLPP can be much more accurately determined as compared to direct visualization of incontinence by the examiner or patient reported incontinence. **When a patient coughs or performs a Valsalva maneuver, fluoroscopy allows the examiner to instantaneously identify incontinence and thus more accurately correlate the VLPP.** The delay of even a fraction of a second when identifying incontinence affects the VLPP value. This is more pronounced for male patients as there is a significant distance between the bladder neck and urethral meatus.

```
┌─────────────────────────────────────────────────────────┐
│ **Scout image**                                         │
│                                                         │
│ • Confirm patient position                              │
│ • Assess for bony abnormalities or residual contrast    │
│   from prior imaging                                    │
└─────────────────────────────────────────────────────────┘
```

```
┌─────────────────────────────────────────────────────────┐
│ **Straining image**                                     │
│                                                         │
│ • Patient to perform Valsalva maneuver and/or cough     │
│ • Assess for stress incontinence, prolapse, or reflux   │
└─────────────────────────────────────────────────────────┘
```

```
┌─────────────────────────────────────────────────────────┐
│ **Voiding cystourethrogram (VCUG)**                     │
│                                                         │
│ • Performed standing (male) or seated (female)          │
│ • Lateral position if urethral pathology suspected      │
│ • Assess for appropriate bladder neck and external      │
│   sphincter function                                    │
└─────────────────────────────────────────────────────────┘
```

```
┌─────────────────────────────────────────────────────────┐
│ **Post-void image**                                     │
│                                                         │
│ • Observe residual contrast in bladder, diverticulum,   │
│   or other area of urinary tract                        │
└─────────────────────────────────────────────────────────┘
```

Fig. 4 Imaging sequence for VUDS

Bladder Outlet Obstruction

Bladder outlet obstruction (BOO) is a straightforward diagnosis when high pressure voiding is in combination with low urine flow; however, the diagnosis is not so easily determined in a female patient or a male patient who has undergone a prostatectomy and also has impaired bladder contractility.

The Use of Fluoroscopy

The simultaneous display of real-time images of the bladder neck and urethra alongside cystometric values of bladder, intra-abdominal, and, in some cases, urethral pressures contributes information on etiology and level of obstruction (stricture, bladder neck dysfunction, prostate outlet obstruction). Specifically, imaging provided by fluoroscopy permits a more accurate determination of the site of obstruction by providing imaging of the bladder neck and urethra while simultaneously measuring bladder pressure and urine flow.

In contrast to many older men in whom prostatic enlargement is often the cause of BOO, young men or men who have had prostate surgery may need a VUDS to evaluate the bladder neck and urethra in order to identify the presence, exact location, and severity of bladder outlet obstruction. Not infrequently a man can continue to have lower urinary tract symptoms (LUTS) such as frequency and urgency following transurethral or open prostatectomy. The resting image provides important information regarding whether the prostatic fossa is appropriately open. Following an adequate transurethral resection of the prostate (TURP), the bladder neck should be open and there should also be a significant defect of the prostatic fossa. In the authors' experience, many men who continue to have LUTS after minimally invasive prostate procedures have a near closed bladder neck and/or a minimal prostatic defect (Fig. 5). In this case the patient should be considered for a TURP. On the contrary, if the bladder neck is open and there is a significant prostatic defect then continued obstruction is unlikely and the concordant bladder pressure tracing can simultaneously assesses for detrusor overactivity as the cause of ongoing LUTS.

During the VCUG portion of the VUDS, the location of any obstruction can be visualized while the associated bladder pressure is evaluated to determine whether obstruction is present and, if so, the degree of obstruction. **A VUDS is invaluable when evaluating a patient for obstruction who has impaired contractility.** In this scenario the diagnosis of obstruction can sometimes only be made by

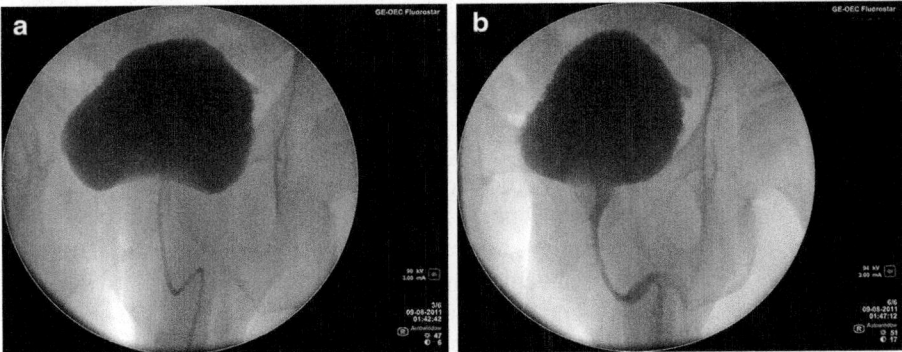

Fig. 5 (**a**) Resting image of a man with continued obstructive symptoms status post laser prostatectomy. The bladder neck is completely closed. (**b**) Voiding film of the same patient. There are multiple diverticulas and there is only a partial defect in the prostatic fossa. The patient subsequently had a transurethral resection of the prostate

visualization of impaired flow of contrast. Again using the post-TURP example, a man who continues to retain urine after TURP is likely still obstructed if contrast is unable to pass the bladder neck or prostatic fossa and the post-TURP defect is minimal, whether he generates a bladder contraction or not.

The ability to diagnose bladder outlet obstruction in women can also be improved with VUDS. Similar to a man with an enlarged prostate, when a woman has advanced vaginal prolapse and difficulty voiding then the diagnosis of BOO is straightforward. On the contrary, the diagnosis of BOO secondary to pelvic floor dysfunction is often confirmed only when the flow of radiographic contrast is shown to be halted at either the bladder neck or external sphincter [13]. Thus, the use of fluoroscopy allows for the correct diagnosis of obstruction in cases when obstruction is not clinically suspected and allows the physician to differentiate between the different categories of obstruction.

Disadvantages of Fluoroscopy

As with all radiographic studies, a disadvantage of fluoroscopy for both patient and operator is radiation exposure. Effective and organ specific doses of ionizing radiation during VUDS can be variable depending on the total time of fluoroscopy use. Nevertheless, studies have shown that patients are exposed to relatively small amounts of radiation during fluoroscopy. One study shows the mean effective dose to be 0.34 mSv and mean fluoroscopy time of 63 s [9]. **Reduction in radiation exposure can be achieved by limiting the time of exposure, maximizing the distance from the radiation source, and shielding. Radiation dose is directly proportional to the time of exposure and to the number of exposures. Thus, exposure time can be minimized by using short bursts of fluoroscopy and using the last image feature.**

Contrast Reactions

The use of a contrast media is necessary for radiographic imaging. Modern injected contrast media are iodine-based. Iodinated contrast comes in two forms: ionic and non-ionic compounds. Non-ionic contrast is significantly more expensive than ionic (approximately 3–5 times the cost); however, non-ionic contrast tends to have less undesirable side effects for the patient. Contrast can be further characterized as being iso-, hyper-, or low-osmolar compared with physiologic osmolality of 300 mOsm/kg of water [14]. Hyperosmolar radiocontrast media can have osomolality as high as 1800 mOsm/kg whereas the low osmolar compounds range from 500 to 600 mOsm/kg. Because these solutions are often more viscous than water, the urodynamics equipment should be calibrated to ensure the accuracy of infused volume, voided volume, and flow rate (See chapter "The Cystometrogram", filling cystometry).

There is no standard practice on contrast use but, in general, lower concentrations are used and they can be further diluted with sterile water to more closely match the viscosity of water.

The physician performing such an evaluation must consider the risks and benefits associated with contrast use. **Adverse side effects and drug reactions have been reported from the intravascular use of contrast media and vary from minor disturbances to severe life threatening situations. Because the contrast is used intravesically rather than intravascularly, these risks are theoretically eliminated.** Premedication strategies exist from H1 receptor blockers to corticosteroid premedication to prevent or reduce the severity of reactions when intravascular contrast is used [15]. Again, theoretically no premedication is necessary when intravesical contrast is used and, in fact, the authors do not premedicate even for patients with known hypersensitivity to intravenous contrast and have not had any untoward reactions.

Troubleshooting

Inability to fill bladder due to severe incompetence of bladder neck

- Bladder neck can be occluded by placing Foley catheter alongside urodynamics catheter and inflating balloon. Gentle traction may also be applied to further occlude the bladder neck.

Urethral catheter not accurately measuring pressure and/or contrast not flowing secondary to kinking of urethral catheter

- Spot fluoroscopy can identify acute angulation of catheter.
- If attempt to reposition catheter does not remedy problem, replace urethral catheter.

Inability to visualize pelvis in obese patient

- Excess soft tissue can significantly impair imaging quality. Image quality can be improved by having patient hold pannus out of x-ray beam field.

Intravesical pressure unchanged throughout study although all catheters functioning

- Catheter tip may be in a diverticulum. If patient has history of diverticulum, withdraw catheter until increase in bladder pressure detected. If there is no history of diverticulum, perform imaging to determine presence.

Patient reports flank pain near beginning of study

- Contrast may be filling ureter. Perform spot fluoroscopy to determine if ureter filling with contrast either due to high bladder pressure or, rarely, urodynamics catheter inadvertently placed in ureter.

Resting film indicates tubular shaped bladder

- Contrast may be filling rectum. Confirm tubing from bottle of contrast attached to bladder catheter and not rectal catheter.

References

1. Winters JC, Dmochowski RR, Goldman HB, Herndon CD, Kobashi KC, Kraus SR, Lemack GE, Nitti VW, Rovner ES, Wein AJ, American Urological A, Society of Urodynamics FPM, Urogenital R. Urodynamic studies in adults: AUA/SUFU guideline. J Urol. 2012;188(6 Suppl):2464–72.
2. Rackley R, Gill B. Urodynamic studies for urinary incontinence medscape. 2013. http://emedicine.medscape.com/article/1988665-overview. Accessed 14 Jul 2014.
3. Bates CP, Whiteside CG, Turner-Warwick R. Synchronous cine-pressure-flow-cysto-urethrography with special reference to stress and urge incontinence. Br J Urol. 1970;42(6):714–23.
4. Enhoerning G, Miller ER, Hinman Jr F. Urethral closure studied with cineroentgenography and simultaneous bladder-urethra pressure recording. Surg Gynecol Obstet. 1964;118:507–16.
5. Pietz M, Gloor E. Fluoroscopy permit requirements. State of California Department of Public Health. 2009. http://www.cdph.ca.gov/pubsforms/forms/Documents/RHB-Fluoroscopy.PDF. Accessed 14 Jul 2014.
6. Geise R, Eubig C, Franz S, Kelsey C, Lieto R, Shaikh N, Wexler M. Managing the use of fluoroscopy in medical institutions, vol. 58. Madison, WI: Medical Physics Publishing; 1998.
7. US Food and Drug Administration. Fluoroscopy. 2014. http://www.fda.gov/radiation-emittingproducts/radiationemittingproductsandprocedures/medicalimaging/medicalx-rays/ucm115354.htm. Accessed 14 Jul 2014.
8. Amis Jr ES, Butler PF, Applegate KE, Birnbaum SB, Brateman LF, Hevezi JM, Mettler FA, Morin RL, Pentecost MJ, Smith GG, Strauss KJ, Zeman RK. American College of Radiology white paper on radiation dose in medicine. J Am Coll Radiol. 2007;4(5):272–84.
9. Giarenis I, Phillips J, Mastoroudes H, Srikrishna S, Robinson D, Lewis C, Cardozo L. Radiation exposure during videourodynamics in women. Int Urogynecol J. 2013;24(9):1547–51.
10. Health Physics Society. Radiation exposure from medical diagnostic imaging procedures. http://hps.org/documents/meddiagimaging.pdf. Accessed 26 Oct 2014.
11. Patel U. Abnormal bladder contour or size. In: Imaging and urodynamics of the lower urinary tract. London: Springer; 2010. p. 57–62.
12. English SF, Amundsen CL, McGuire EJ. Bladder neck competency at rest in women with incontinence. J Urol. 1999;161(2):578–80.
13. Nitti VW, Tu LM, Gitlin J. Diagnosing bladder outlet obstruction in women. J Urol. 1999;161(5):1535–40.
14. American College of Radiology. ACR manual on contrast media, version 9. http://www.acr.org/~/media/ACR/Documents/PDF/QualitySafety/Resources/Contrast%20Manual/2013_Contrast_Media.pdf. Accessed 26 Oct 2001.
15. Wittbrodt ET, Spinler SA. Prevention of anaphylactoid reactions in high-risk patients receiving radiographic contrast media. Ann Pharmacother. 1994;28(2):236–41.

Putting It All Together: Practical Advice on Clinical Urodynamics

Julian Wan and John T. Stoffel

Introduction

Urodynamics to be meaningful in a clinical sense must be deployed in the real world. The real world application however often requires accommodation and adjustment of clinical routines. It also requires some forethought and planning. The following chapter covers some of these practical aspects of real world urodynamics. Some patience is required when implementing urodynamics especially into an already established practice.

Tests and Simulations

Urodynamics are among the most useful clinical tests for the urologists but for new users they can be confusing and daunting at times. They are not quite full blown procedures such as a cystoscopy but are not non-invasive. As clinical tools they should not be viewed any differently than other clinical tests we regularly order and interpret. Some tests which we use are very straightforward. When abnormal they

---

J. Wan, M.D., F.A.A.P. (✉)
Division of Pediatric Urology, Department of Urology, C.S. Mott Children's and Von Voigtlander Women's Hospital, 3875 Taubman Center, SPC 5330, 1500 East Medical Center Drive, Ann Arbor, MI 48109-5330, USA
e-mail: juliwan@umich.edu

J.T. Stoffel, M.D.
Division of Neurourology and Pelvic Reconstructive Surgery, Department of Urology, University of Michigan Medical Center, 3875 Taubman Center, SPC 5330, 1500 East Medical Center Drive, Ann Arbor, MI 48109-5330, USA
e-mail: jstoffel@med.umich.edu

© Springer International Publishing Switzerland 2016
A.C. Peterson, M.O. Fraser (eds.), *Practical Urodynamics for the Clinician*,
DOI 10.1007/978-3-319-20834-3_9

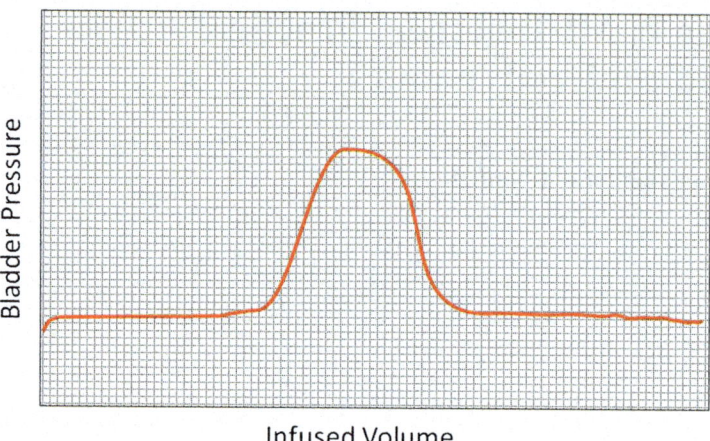

Fig. 1 Example of a cystometric tracing. It could be due to pathology, a test artifact or normal activity. Clinical context is needed

point to a specific pathology. The serum sodium level, for example, when low suggests hyponatremia and possible fluid overload. The chest x-ray which shows the edges of the pleura away from the chest wall points to a pneumothorax. Most tests, however, have practical limits and to be truly useful they require clinical context to avoid artifacts and incorrect interpretation. A patient with severe hyperglycemia-such as seen in diabetic ketoacidosis can have a falsely low serum sodium concentration due to an artifact in testing relating to the extracellular shifts of water [1, 2].

Part of the challenge for new users is that urodynamics are not specific like otherdiagnostic testsand the results are dependent on clinical context. It is helpful to think of findings on urodynamics as one of three possibilities. First, a finding can represent a pathological result which is indicative of a presence of some disease state or abnormality. For example, EMG changes during voiding in Fig. 1 can represent neurogenic voiding dysfunction. Second, the urodynamic finding can also be an artifact related to normal patient activity or a limitation of the test. The cystometrogram for example may show a rise in bladder pressure (see Fig. 1). But this finding could also be from the patient adjusting her position and pressing down on her pelvis. In this scenario, the "surge" seen on the CMG actually represents the external pressure of her abdominal contents shifting down on the bladder. Third, a finding on urodynamics can represent normal function for the context of the study. For example, a nervous patient whose bladder is filled quickly will rapidly reach functional capacity and report a strong desire to void. The contraction of the bladder in this context represents normal physiology.

In summary, testing needs clinical context to have clinical meaning. Accurate interpretation of urodynamics demands knowledge oftheclinical situation and the circumstances of testing, otherwise one cannot be sure of the meaning of the results.

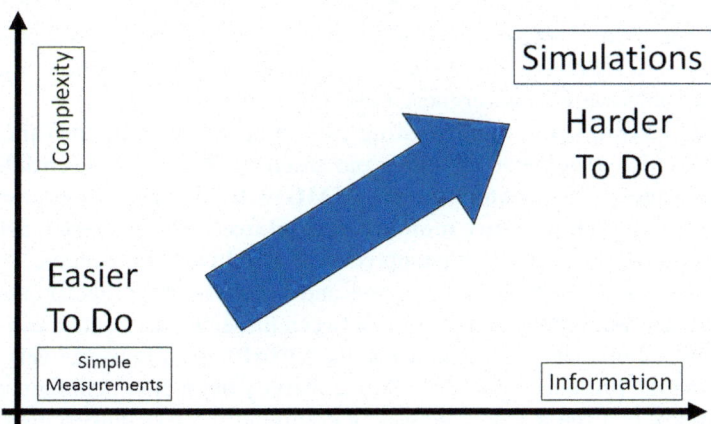

Fig. 2 The relationship between complexity and information. The simpler and easier to do measurements such as the uroflow and post-void residual (*lower left hand corner*) are robust but do not provide very much information. The more complex studies (*upper right hand corner*) such as the pressure-flow and Valsalva leak point pressure study provide much more information but are harder to execute. In general, the more complex the study, the more complete the simulation of the clinical question

The tests themselves vary in complexity. Some are simple measurements of a urologic parameter. Others are more complex recreations or simulations of a specific clinical situation. The simpler tests are easier to perform and replicate. The more complex tests take more time, energy and resources but can yield a more complete answer. The price for this information however is the potential for more complex artifacts. In general, tests which are simple measurements are easy to do but provide less information. More complex simulations provide much more data and a more complete picture of the patient at the cost of greater complexity and difficulty in performance (see Fig. 2). Much of the art of using urodynamics comes from applying the appropriately level of complexity to solve the clinical question.

Simple urodynamic measurements include the uroflow and post-void residual. The former is nearly ubiquitous in all urology offices and measures how fast urine is voided from the bladder. **As a screening test the uroflow is very helpful but it cannot easily differentiate between different pathophysiologies when it is abnormal**. Is a poor uroflow result due to a weak detrusor or is there some outlet obstruction? Post void residual is typically obtained today using a small dedicated ultrasound device (BladderScan® [3]) although sterile catheterization is still used. Like the uroflow the post-void residual when normal is very helpful in that it suggest complete emptying is occurring. This conclusion can then be used to infer (assuming the absence of any other findings) that the bladder and urethra can empty effectively in an unimpeded normal fashion. **Like the uroflow, when the post-void residual is abnormal it is unclear as to why.** Is it due to a urethral stricture or prostatic enlargement? Could it be an areflexic hypoactive bladder? To further complicate interpretations, true ranges of normal values of post void residuals have not been completely validated. These simple parameter tests while useful, easy to perform and reliable cannot answer these more involved questions.

The next level of urodynamic testing encompasses the more advanced measurements which track two or more parameters. They are essentially small scale simulations. Thecystometrogram (CMG)with or without electromyography, rectal or vaginal pressure monitoring, and urethral pressure tracking are examples. The CMG, often the unappreciated workhorse urodynamic test tracks two parameters—infused bladder volume and intravesical storage pressure. It is excellent at determining the relationship between these two parameters expressed as the bladder compliance (mathematically as $\Delta V/\Delta P$). It is however very poor in documenting the presence or absence of overactivity in the non-neurogenic patient. It is a paradox that the act of testing may confound the test. Superficially it may seem that the CMG would be ideal for this purpose since it seems to simulate the situation many patients with bladder overactivity (OAB) encounter—an unexpected sense of urgency during routine bladder filling. Yet, in practice the act of testing often yields a high false negative result, making it practically useless as a screening test for this purpose [4]. The solution to this paradox lies in the understanding that the act of testing does not in fact recreate a true simulation of the clinical circumstance. The typical overactive adult patient reports being caught off guard with a sudden feeling of urgency or even urge incontinence. During testing the patient is awake, catheterized and is now consciously focused on the bladder, its sensations and the pelvis in general. This is not the typical clinical scenario when the patient's mind is busy with the daily routines of life; it is not focused on the bladder. The act of testing is creating an artificial situation. Rather than the more accurate depiction with a distracted patient, the test creates a misleading situation where the patient is completely focused on the bladder. During the test, this focus helps prevent the occurrence of the over activity. But this level of bladder focus is not possible practically for most patients who are trying to carry on with their lives. For this reason some researchers have advocated using continuous pressure monitoring with ambulatory urodynamics if testing is truly needed or simply treating symptomatically without using urodynamics if simple OAB is suspected (See chapter "Ambulatory Urodynamics") [5, 6]. **The highest level of urodynamic simulation combines several parameters and adds the patient's cooperation to recreate the events and forces leading to the patient's symptoms.** Two common situations include the man who is having difficulty voiding and the woman with intermittent incontinence which may be related to stress. The best known of these are the pressure flow and stress incontinence tests which are done commonly with fluoroscopy. These tests track the infused bladder volume,intravesical storage and voiding pressures, coordination of the bladder neck and sphincter as well as urinary flow and leakage. The key factor is that at an appropriate point when the bladder is filled to the level that approximates the usual clinical situation, the patient is asked to volitionally void or bear down and try to recreate the leakage or obstruction. We can visualize and note at what volume and how much pressure (measured in cm H_2O) it takes to induce leakage or how much pressure it takes to drive urine across the obstructive prostatic hypertrophy. The study therefore not only should capture the event, but it also allows us to quantify the forces involved thereby revealing objective measurements which can be used to compare treatment results and efficacy.

The Urodynamic Laboratory

The distinction between urodynamic tests is not merely an academic or intellectual one. They become important when one considers setting up an urodynamic laboratory. For simple measurements one can easily set up the lab so the tests can be done by the support staff. The instructions and set ups are simple and require no direct provider supervision. It becomes trickier with the more complex studies. Basically these studies can be one of two ways. They can be done by the urologist with assistance from his support staff or in some cases they can be done completely by the assistants themselves and read by the urologist after testing is completed. There are nurses, physician assistants and medical assistants who are quite skillful, well trained and fully capable of performing even the most complicated studies. **If the urologist is going to be present at each test then the issues about clinical context discussed earlier is still important. The urologist is physically present and can talk with the patient directly and can be assured that the desired simulation is recreated. If the urologist will not be present during the study and it is the plan to set up a laboratory as a unit that functions without the provider's direct participation in the testing process, it is critical that the team doing the studies have very clear communication with the urologist who will be interpreting the results and an understanding about which clinical questions need to be addressed during testing.**

Simply having the team undergo a training course is not sufficient. After 20 years of teaching courses to urologists who are trying to incorporate urodynamics into their daily clinical practice, **the failure to recognize the need to establish a consistent common understanding among all of the team members including the urologist, is the primary cause of most unsuccessful efforts to implement urodynamics into an existing practice.** Lacking a clear grasp of the aim of the study and what exactly the urologist is seeking to discover the team can become unsure and may not provide the needed information or do studies which are unnecessary out of fear of overlooking something. The urologist can become frustrated at the output being received and loses confidence in the team and the utility of the tests. The urologist who will be interpreting the results and the team performing the test must have a shared understanding of how the tests are done and how the results are recorded and presented. Ideally the team and the urologist should do a series of tests together over 6–12 months so that they develop the same understanding of how the tests are conducted, the terminology and have an established protocol of how the data are stored and displayed. The ICS best urodynamic practices document is a helpful aid in establishing standardized practices for urologist and testing team [6]. They will then have a common set of experiences of dealing with artifacts, how the data are reported out and interpreted. Seemingly minor considerations such as the exact layout of the room, where commonly used items are stored, and the patient flow should be worked out in details. True team work, a clear understanding and open communication are needed to make this type of set-up work.

Fluoroscopy

General Considerations

The discussion of the utility of fluoroscopy in urodynamics is not one of whether there is a benefit but rather one of whether the benefits justify the additional costs and effort. When considering cost it must be understood that this cost is not limited to just the fluoroscopy machine itself (See chapter "The Use of Fluoroscopy"). It must also include the cost of operation, maintenance, safety requirements and certification. A basic c-arm style fluoroscopy unit can be acquired new, used or refurbished from between $10,000 to $150,000 depending on the make, model and features (Block Imaging [7]). In addition there are the costs of safety accessories such as lead aprons, shields, and glasses. Each person who is working with the device will need to be trained and must achieve and maintain some level of certification for radiation safety. Monitoring is almost always necessary and typically is done with a system of regular dosimetry badge readings. The particular details and costs will of course vary with the region and institution but the actual lease or purchase price of the machine may only be a small fraction of the total cost over time.

The physical plant where the fluoroscopy will be used needs to be considered. Some new facilities have rooms which are pre-built to be x-ray imaging rooms, but others especially when retrofitting an existing clinical space will require additional shielding. Placement of the machine may also alter how the room will be outfitted with radio-opaque material. In the USA there is no national standard and each state has its own variations. In some states this is handled by the state's department of health whereas others have distinct radiology departments. For example, the State of Michigan handles these matters through the Department of Licensing and Regulatory Affairs within a Radiation Safety Section [8]. Typically there are minimal thickness levels of lead or equivalent material in the walls, floor and ceilings with specified levels of exposure. Positioning of the device is a critical factor. Rooms closer to public areas require higher minimal distances and radio-opacity ratings depending on the potential exposure risk. Devices such as c-arm machines which can project radiation over a wide arc increase the at-risk area. These would in turn increase the separation distances and radio-opacity requirements when compared to a fixed machine aiming downwards toward the ground. Because of the wide regional variation, a careful review of the local rules and regulation is necessary when contemplating the addition of fluoroscopy [8]. The different options of business models for medical equipment purchase, lease and rental offers potential cost savings. Beyond the scope of this chapter for more detail discussion, these considerations and the tax effects of equipment depreciation all should be considered when weighing the options. Finally another approach is to lease or rent a fully equipped licensed imaging suite. Some imaging services and centers allow outside qualified practitioners to arrange a long term lease or rent as needed their imaging suites. This would allow an otherwise fallow room to be productive. The newer portable urodynamic units make it easy to bring the needed equipment to the imaging suite. When one is weighing the benefits of using fluoroscopy, a careful analysis of the options and total costs is necessary. Fundamentally does the practice expect to see enough patients who would benefit from having fluoroscopy to warrant the financial outlay?

Benefits

The principalbenefitsoffered by the use of fluoroscopy are improved efficiency of work up and more diagnosis specific information. For patients in whom there is a concern about vesicoureteral reflux, diverticuli, or who had prior complex reconstructions or atypical bladder anatomy, fluoroscopy during urodynamics obviates the need to perform a separate VCUG or cystogram. Incidental information can be gathered about important complementary conditions such as constipation and orthopedic fractures. Constipation and impacted stool are easy to see and for some patients prove more accurate than their self-reporting.

The bladder neck and urethral status are easy to visualize. An open bladder neck at rest, a kinked or acutely suspended urethra after a failed pubovaginal sling or needle suspension procedure, dysfunctional proximal urethral, urethral strictures and the presence and location of radio-opaque implanted structures are all easy to see. Genital prolapse can be seen and the effect of repositioning the bladder neck and urethra back into a normal position (with help of a pessary or folded gauze roll) can be visualized. The images once captured can also be shown to the patients and families and helps make the process of explaining the risks and benefits of any procedure easier. This is especially true when dealing with complications of an earlier failed operation. Finally, fluoro-urodynamics is particularly useful for patients who have complex anatomy because of a concomitant finding such as a large diverticulum, severe vesicoureteral reflux or after prior surgery especially reconstructions such as enteroaugmentation, continent catheterizable stoma, or neobladder. The clinician is granted the opportunity to fill the system and be certain that all of the various compartments and segments are indeed filled and correlate these observations with storage pressure readings. For example, a neurogenic patient with severe vesicoureteral reflux or diverticulum, failed repair of the reflux by reimplantion or excision of the diverticulum may inadvertently drastically decrease the important part of the patient's storage capacity. The patient may have been actually venting high storage pressure into the tortuous refluxing ureters or into the large diverticulum (see Figs. 3 and 4). Failing to recognize this possibility may lead to later renal deterioration due to high post-operative storage pressures. Similarly if after a complex surgery which continues to have issues, being able to link storage pressures with the true state of filling can be crucial. For example, a neurogenic patient continues to have signs and symptoms consistent with hyperreflexic contractions despite what was reported as being an ileal augmentation cystoplasty. The patient comes in for a second opinion with spurting leakage and seemingly a low functional capacity. A simple plain cystogram would show the contractions at the lower than expected volumes but a fluorourodynamic study would reveal that the anastomosis of the ileal segment had contracted giving a "dumb bell" shaped augmentation—essentially neutralizing the potential benefit of the original procedure.

Complex Cystometrogram

The term complex cystometrogram is given to a combination of the basic cystometrogram (CMG) with an additional component. Typically this would be an EMG, abdominal pressure through a rectal or vaginal balloon, or fluoroscopy.

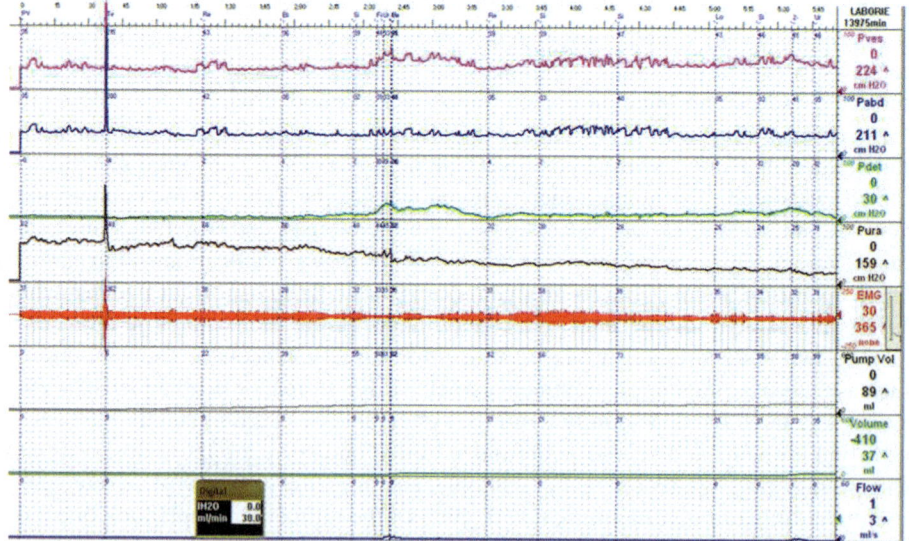

Fig. 3 Is this cystometrogram tracing worrisome? The bladder pressure curve seems flat

Reflux at low volumes prevents rise in CMG pressure

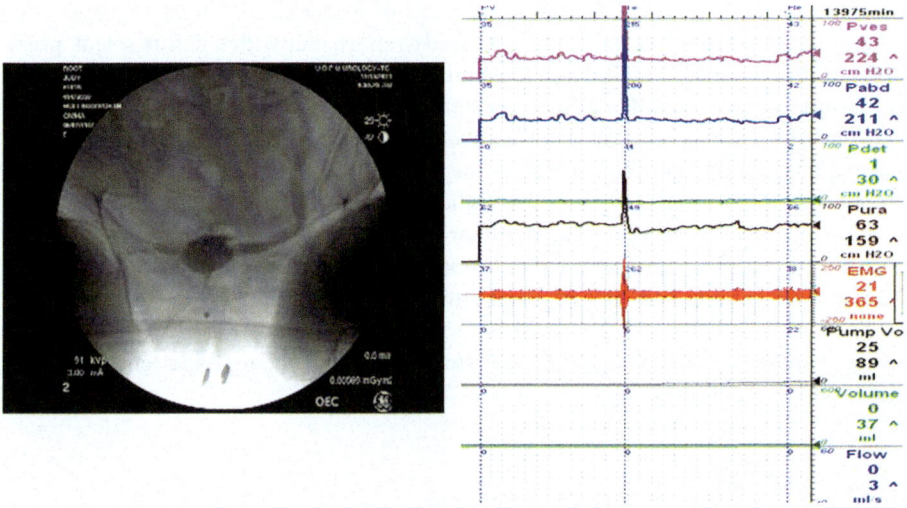

Fig. 4 Simultaneous fluoroscopy shows that the bladder pressure curve is being artificially kept flat because of high grade vesicoureteral reflux. The reflux vents the pressure into the upper tracts. Without fluoroscopy this would be missed

The cystometrogram yields information about bladder compliance and the added component gives some complementary data. The EMG can show if the patient has coordinated activity or is experiencing detrusor sphincter dyssynergia. The abdominal pressure can help determine the effect of external forces (which can be simulated using a Valsalva maneuver) on the continence mechanism of the bladder neck and proximal urethra. Finally fluoroscopy as noted above yields potentially a whole host of observations concerning the bladder, bladder neck and other structures; it visually relates storage pressure findings with what is going on with lower urinary tract.

While it is always desirable economically and in terms of efficiency to only order as much testing as necessary, it may be hard to anticipate practically which components one should have in the complex cystometrogram. One could simply "doing everything" and have all patients undergo a full urodynamic study with fluoroscopy, multi-channel (bladder, urethra) monitoring, with uroflowmetry, EMG and abdominal subtraction. While this "do everything" approach certainly can work it is wasteful of time, resources and money. This segues naturally to the concept of tailoring studies to the specific clinical question.

A CMG reveals not only bladder compliance at a fixed point in time but over a complete cycle from empty to full functional volume. Given time and continued filling everybody, even those with normal bladders, will exhaust the compliance of their reservoirs, but usually this theoretical limit is never reached practically. Knowing the practical functional volume and the compliance curve to that point is what is clinically relevant. Consider the case of a spinal cord injury patient who undergoes a cystometrogram study. The study reports out with a detrusor leak point pressure of 55 cm H_2O at 700 ml. The high detrusor leak point pressure is certainly worrisome since it is well over the generally accepted "red line" limit of 40 cm H_2O discovered by McGuire et al. [9]. However, when one looks at the cathing diary of this patient and the compliance curve one sees that this person normally caths and empties at or before 450 ml, and the highest storage pressure experienced at these volumes is only 15 cm H_2O. The detrusor leak point pressure in this case while an accurate reading is moot because that is not what the patient practically experiences. Keeping with the notion that an ideal study simulates the clinical question being posed, in this case the clinical question is not what is the detrusor leak point pressure but rather what is the intravesical storage pressure being experienced by this patient during everyday life.

Tailoring the Study for Specific Clinical Questions

Neurogenic Bladder Patients

For neurogenic bladderpatients the key parameters being evaluated are the storage pressure, the status of the bladder neck, the coordination of bladder and sphincter, and whether reflux is present [15]. The normal bladder depends on an intact neural system to coordinate the detrusor and sphincter as well as modulate bladder relaxation during filling. Patients with neurogenic bladders often suffer from changes in these behaviors. **Urodynamic testing not only helps monitor for changes but also could help pre-empt and prevent future problems.** For example, many patients with spina bifida develop neurogenic bladders which require regular pressure monitoring. They also can have open bladder necks which leak passively and prevent them from becoming socially dry between intermittent catheterization. Were one to simple do a bladder neck continence procedure or place a pubovaginal/prostatic sling without first checking on bladder compliance, it potentially places the patient at serious risk for future bladder and renal deterioration if the patient has underlying low bladder compliance. The open bladder neck allowed easy leakage and venting of the bladder thereby keeping bladder storage pressures low. After the continence procedure, this "safety valve" effect is gone and very high and damaging storage pressures (>40 cm H_2O) can develop [10, 11]. This concern has also been seen in patients with occult low compliance who have had placement of an artificial urinary sphincter [12].

Non-neurogenic Incontinent Patients

For non-neurogenic incontinent patients the emphasis is to recreate the circumstances of incontinence thereby creating the most accurate simulation of what is happening when wetting occurs. If the patient reports wetting with straining when upright, the study should ideally be done with the patient in an upright or at least a seated posture and ideally with fluoroscopy either in a coronal or saggital view. This would better simulate the effect of having the peritoneal contents on the bladder and make the transmission of any abdominal pressure more effective and realistic. For this situation the use of a rectal or vaginal catheter is necessary. It would help objectively measure the abdominal pressure and allow through the use of digital subtraction an accurate measure of the vesical contribution. The intravesical pressure being the sum of the pressure from the bladder and the transmitted pressure from the abdomen, simply subtracting the data from the rectal or vaginal catheter from the intravesical pressure yields the vesical contribution. Being able to measure the peritoneal component also allows an opportunity to be sure the simulation is accurate. The process of having an urodynamic study can be embarrassing and having a variety of catheters in the urethra, rectum or vagina may make it hard for many to fully bear down and recreate the pressures and forces which they experience when they wet in real life. When one is performing these tests such as the Valsalva Leak Point Pressure one can visualize whether the effort is a realistic one [13, 14]. For most adults, a pressure up to 100 cm H_2O would be a reasonable effort. If the effort is weak, it may not fully stress the system and a false negative result may occur. Under fluoroscopy the effect of genital prolapse can be seen and one can temporarily minimize the effect with a pessary or by placing a sponge into the vagina and retesting.

References

1. Katz MA. Hyperglycemia-induced hyponatremia calculation of expected serum sodium depression. NEJM. 1973;289(16):843–4.
2. Hillier TA, Abbott RD, Barrett EJ. Hyponatremia: evaluating the correction factor for hyperglycemia. Am J Med. 1999;106(4):399–403.
3. BladderScan®, Verathon Inc., Bothell, WA, USA
4. Daan NM, Schweitzer KM, van der Vaart CH. Associations between subjective bladder symptoms and objective parameters on bladder diary and filling cystometry. Int Urogynecol J. 2012; 23(11):1619–24.
5. van Waalwijk van Doorn ES, Meier AH, Ambergen AW, Janknegt RA. Ambulatory urodynamics: extramural testing of the lower and upper urinary tract by Holter monitoring of cystometrogram, uroflowmetry, and renal pelvic pressures. Urol Clin North Am. 1996;23:345–71.
6. Swithinbank LV, James M, Shepherd A, Abrams P. Role of ambulatory urodynamics monitoring in clinical urological practice. Neurourol Urodyn. 1999;20:249–57.
7. Block Imaging website. 2014. http://info.blockimaging.com/bid/70225/Awesome-C-Arm-Price-Infographic-Compare-C-Arm-Machine-Prices. Retrieved 1 Sept 2014.

8. State of Michigan Department of Licensing and Regulatory Affairs within a Radiation Safety Section websit. 2014. http://www.michigan.gov/lara/0,4601,7-154-61256_11407_35791---,00.html. Retrieved 1 Sept 2014.
9. McGuire EJ, Woodside JR, Borden TA, Weiss RM. Prognostic value of urodynamic testing in myelodysplastic patients. J Urol. 1981;126(2):205–9.
10. Ghoniem GM, Bloom DA, McGuire EJ, Stewart KL. Bladder compliance in meningomyelocele children. J Urol. 1989;141:1404–6.
11. Gormley EA, Bloom DA, McGuire EJ, Ritchey ML. Pubovaginal slings for the management of urinary incontinence in female adolescents. J Urol. 1994;152:822–5.
12. Roth DR, Vyas PR, Kroovand RL, Perlmutter AD. Urinary tract deterioration associated with the artificial urinary sphincter. J Urol. 1986;135(3):528–30.
13. Wan J, McGuire EJ, Bloom DA, Ritchey ML. The treatment of urinary incontinence in children using glutaraldehyde cross-linked collagen. J Urol. 1992;148(1):127–30.
14. McGuire EJ, Cespedes RD, O'Connell HE. Leak-point pressures. Urol Clin North Am. 1996;23(2):253–62.
15. Schafer W, Abrams P, Liao L, Anders M, Pesce F, Spangbert A, Sterling AM, Zinner NR, van Kerrebroeck P. Good urodynamic practices: uroflowmetry, filling cystometry and pressure-flow studies. Neurourol Urodyn. 2002;21:261–74.

Nomograms

David Jiang and Jennifer Tash Anger

Introduction

Pressure-flow urodynamic studies have been used to diagnose bladder outlet obstruction in both men and women for many years. Classically, high-pressure, low flow is typical of bladder outlet obstruction; however, the exact combination of pressure-flow at which obstruction should be diagnosed has not been clearly established. **A pressure-flow nomogram is a useful graphic and computational tool that aids in the proper identification and differentiation of those who have true bladder outlet obstruction from those who have other flow issues such as underactive detrusor function, or a combination of both. Additionally, nomograms allow us to diagnose bladder outlet obstruction in a reproducible manner by using concrete inputs obtained from the urodynamics study.** Using detrusor pressure at peak flow and the peak flow rate, obtained from urodynamic studies, we can estimate the etiology of the urinary dysfunction. Several nomograms have been established and accepted for use in men (Abrams-Griffiths nomogram, Schäfer nomogram, and ICS nomogram); The Blaivas-Groutz nomogram has been established for women.

D. Jiang, M.D., M.Sc.
Oregon Health and Science University, Department of Urology, Portland, OR, USA
e-mail: jianda@ohsu.edu

J.T. Anger, M.D., M.P.H. (✉)
Division of Urology, Department of Surgery, Cedars-Sinai Medical Center,
99 N. La Cienaga Blvd., #307, Beverly Hills, CA 90211, USA
e-mail: Jennifer.anger@cshs.org

Abrams-Griffiths Nomogram

Paul Abrams and Derek Griffiths collaborated together in 1979 at the Ham Green Hospital in Bristol to construct the Abrams-Griffiths nomogram. Dr. Abrams introduced the term "Lower Urinary Tract Symptoms (LUTS)" in 1994 and, with Alan Wein, the term "Overactive Bladder (OAB) in 1996. Dr. Griffiths has a strong background in physics; he worked closely with Paul Abrams and Werner Schäfer to explore the intricacies of voiding dysfunction. The Abrams-Griffiths nomogram was developed from pressure-flow studies of 117 men age 55 and older who were evaluated for possible benign prostatic hyperplasia. The investigators measured various parameters of the voiding cycle. They determined the urethral closure pressure profile and filling cystometry; additionally they measured the intravesical pressure, rectal pressure, and volume voided during micturition. A pressure-flow plot was generated from the data. Prior to this study, it was suggested that, in unobstructed states, the mean slope (change in pressure/change in flow) of the pressure-flow plot (after the fast initial rise in flow rate) is less than 2 cm $H_2O/ml/s$ and the detrusor pressure as flow ceases at the end of voiding is 40 cm $H_2O/ml/s$ or less. Fifteen of the patients eventually received simple prostatectomy; Abrams and Griffiths measured their voiding cycle parameters 3 months after surgery. The authors inserted all the data points on the pressure-flow plot and found that there were clusters of patients who were obstructed on the upper side of the plot and the non-obstructed patients on the lower side. They generated a nomogram based on this data.

The nomogram plot is based on the detrusor pressure at maximum flow as well as the maximum flow rate (Fig. 1a). **From this plot, three zones separate obstructed, unobstructed, and equivocal result. By entering the detrusor pressure at the maximum flow ($P_{detQmax}$) and the maximum flow (Q_{max}) of a patient's urodynamic study, one can determine if the patient has bladder outlet obstruction** [1].

The Abrams-Griffiths nomogram boundaries were created by a combination of clinical and theoretical observations. Patients had been evaluated clinically prior to the pressure flow study and determined to have obstruction. For those patients who fall in the equivocal region, further analysis based on the traditional criteria can be performed to determine whether the patient is obstructed or not. A pressure-flow curve of the complete micturition is used in this case. If the mean slope of the pressure-flow plot is less than 2 cm $H_2O/ml/s$ and the minimal voiding detrusor pressure is less than 40 cm H_2O, then the bladder outlet is unobstructed (Fig. 1b). Conversely, either a slope greater than 2 cm $H_2O/ml/s$ (Fig. 1c) or a minimal voiding detrusor pressure greater than 40 cm H_2O (Fig. 1d) indicates a bladder outlet obstruction. Using this method, all patients can be classified as obstructed or unobstructed.

The nomogram has been used to study outcomes of prostatectomy in 123 patients [2]. In this prospective study, patients were selected for prostatectomy based on clinical symptom score, but the results of the pressure-flow studies were blinded both pre- and post-operatively (at 6 months after surgery). Thirty-six out of 123 patients were found to be "unobstructed" based on the Abrams-Griffiths nomogram

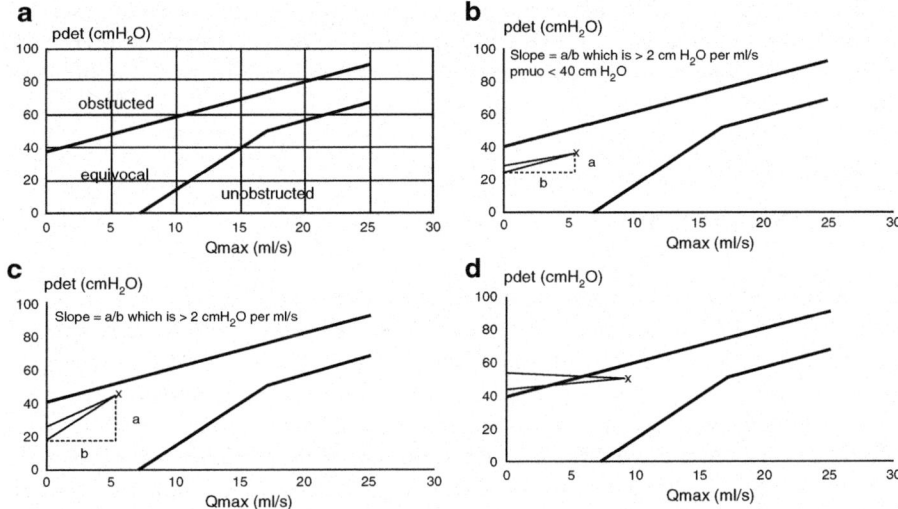

Fig. 1 (a) Abrams-Griffiths nomogram. Plot uses detrusor pressure at maximum urinary flow and maximum urinary flow rate. Reproduced from Lim CS and Abrams P. The Abrams-Griffith nomogram. *World J Urol.* 1995;13:35, with permission of Springer. (**b**) Initially equivocal on the Abrams-Griffiths nomogram further analyzed as an unobstructed pattern. Slope ≤ 2 cm H_2O/ml/s and minimal voiding detrusor pressure ≤ 40 cm H_2O. (**c**) Initially equivocal on the Abrams-Griffiths nomogram further analyzed as obstructed pattern because slope >2 cm H_2O/ml/s. (**d**) Initially equivocal on the Abrams-Griffiths nomogram further analyzed as obstructed pattern because minimal voiding pressure >40 cm H_2O

pre-operatively; unsurprisingly, their post-operative pressure-flow curve remained in the unobstructed category. In the 87 patients found to be "obstructed" pre-operatively, their pressure-flow parameters after prostatectomy improved significantly and were categorized as unobstructed. The success rate as measured by severity of symptoms was 93.1 % in the obstructed group, but only 77.8 % in the unobstructed group. **The Abrams-Griffiths nomogram not only helps determine obstructed from unobstructed patients but also provides information on the outcome of the operation as those who were categorized as obstructed pre-operatively had a more significant positive clinical outcome.** The use of the Abrams-Griffiths nomogram has also been validated for transurethral resection of prostate [3]. Similar to Jensen's group, Rollema and Mastrigt observed that patients who were previously obstructed according to the nomogram had improved pressure-flow parameters after the transurethral resection of the prostate. They also found that patients who were categorized as unobstructed prior to surgery had a less dramatic improvement in voiding symptoms compared those who were categorized as obstructed. It is believed that, in those patients who are symptomatic but have an unobstructed pressure-flow curve, the problem is impaired detrusor contractility and surgery for bladder outlet obstruction will not improve their symptoms. They suggest using the Abrams-Griffiths nomogram as possible method to screen patients prior to surgery.

The Abrams-Griffiths nomogram is therefore useful for the diagnosis of bladder outlet obstruction. Specifically, it is helpful to predict which men with bladder outlet obstruction from enlarged prostates will benefit from surgical intervention.

Schäfer Nomogram

Werner Schäfer initially studied aeronautical and spacecraft engineering from the Aachen University in Germany. His background in physics and biomedical engineering was instrumental in his detailed analysis of voiding function. He developed a nomogram in 1990 based on the concept that flow of urine is initiated when the pressure from the bladder is equal to or slightly exceeds the intrinsic urethral pressure. The collapsed urethra differs from a rigid pipe in that intraluminal pressure is required to open the lumen before flow can occur. **The pressure point where the urethra opens to allow micturition is also called the*urethral opening pressure*. A special feature of flow in a collapsible and distensible tube, like the urethra, is that the pressure-flow relation can be controlled by a single small segment acting as a flow-controlling zone.** Under physiologic conditions, this zone is at the pelvic floor level; however in pathological outflow conditions, the obstruction itself takes over the role of the flow-controlling zone. As the bladder pressure increases from the urethral opening pressure, the urethra opens and the rate of flow increases sharply. Therefore, by graphing the detrusor pressure vs. flow rate during a course of micturition, one can obtain the urethral resistance to flow (Fig. 2).

Changes in lumen size and opening pressure can affect the pressure-flow curve separately, thus creating different forms of obstruction: constrictive or compressive. Constrictive obstruction can be exemplified by urethral stricture disease; compressive obstruction is typically seen in benign prostatic hyperplasia. These can be differentiated using urodynamics studies. With a constrictive obstruction, micturition can be initiated and maintained with a normal low pressure, but the energy balance during the mid-flow is unfavorable. In a compressive obstruction, the increased energy demand is not just limited to the mid-flow but also for the initiation and termination of micturition. The higher urethral opening pressure requires a prolonged isovolumetric contraction phase before flow can start and requires a proportionately higher minimum muscle power to maintain flow. The difference in minimum voiding power explains why large residual urine volumes are common in compressive obstructions but rare in constrictive obstructions. For ease of description and understanding, the curve can be rotated to have the flow rate on the Y-axis and detrusor pressure on the X-axis. The flow-pressure plot can show complex patterns; however it is most important to determine the lowest resistance since this is closely related to bladder outlet morphology. **The line generated on the flow-pressure plot is a simple quadratic shape, which is referred to as the*passive urethral resistance relation* (PURR).** The slope and position of the passive urethral resistance relation can provide information about the opening pressure and the effective lumen size of the flow. Obstruction caused by benign prostatic hyperplasia

Fig. 2 Detrusor pressure vs. flow rate curves. Reproduced from Blaivas J. Multichannel urodynamic studies. *Urol.* 1984;23:421–438, with permission of Elsevier. (**a**) Normal: flow is initiated at a pressure of 50 cm H$_2$O, and flow rate increases to almost 20 ml/s with no further appreciable rise in pressure. (**b**) Bladder outlet obstruction: flow is not initiated until detrusor pressure of 100 cm H$_2$O and, despite further rise in detrusor pressure, maximum flow attains only 6 ml/s

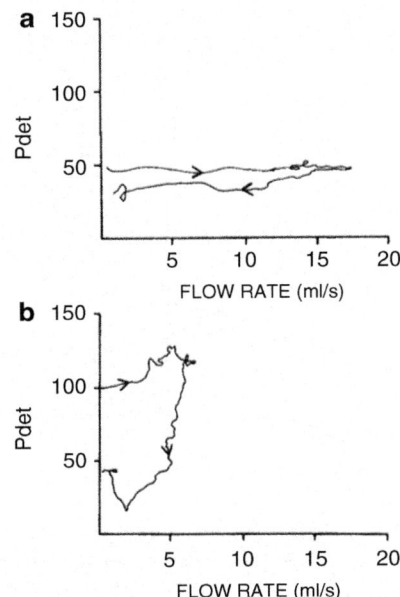

has a *compressive* curve and shifts the micturition curve further to the right on the flow vs. pressure diagram, whereas urethral strictures have *constrictive* curves and are "flat" (Fig. 3).

The linearized passive urethral relation curve (linPURR) is a derivative of the passive urethral resistance relation curve [4]. Flow rate is measured on the Y-axis and the detrusor pressure on the X-axis. **The Schäfer nomogram is divided into seven zones (0–VI) corresponding to increasing grades of obstruction, where 0–I (unobstructed), zone II (equivocal or mild obstruction), zones III–VI (more severe grades of obstruction). There are also four zones for roughly estimating detrusor contraction from very weak to strong, which is based on the point of maximum flow and the associated detrusor pressure** (Fig. 3).

The first value obtained is the lowest detrusor pressure value at which urine starts or stops. Schäfer suggests making appropriate corrections for the flow rate delay and for potential inaccuracies of the flowmeter when the flow starts or ends during rapid detrusor pressure changes. Prostatic obstruction is generally located at the proximal urethra. Therefore, it is reasonable to cut off the last few milliliters (approximately 5 ml) accumulating in the flowmeter at very low flow rate, around 2 ml/s, before the flow finally ceases. These last few drops are more likely to originate from draining of the distal urethra than from real flow through the prostatic obstruction. The second value obtained is the pressure at the maximum flow rate ($P_{detQmax}$), which according to Schäfer, is easier to obtain than the lowest detrusor pressure at the start or stop of flow. Those two points can then be plotted on a pressure-flow graph and connected via a straight line. That line can be measured against the Schäfer nomogram. The shape of the line and the distance on the X-axis can determine

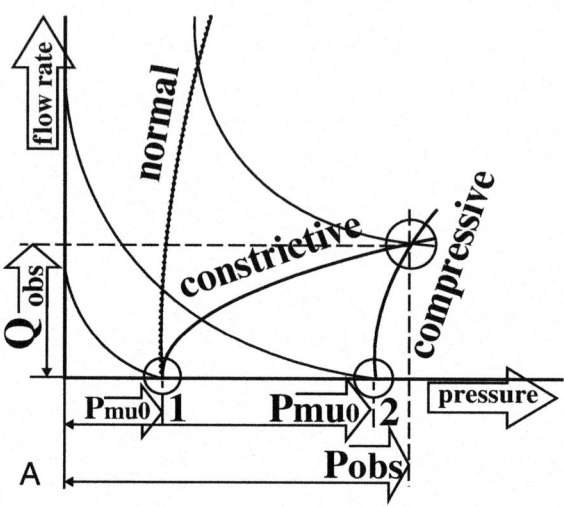

Fig. 3 Passive urethral resistance relation. Specific types of obstruction are demonstrated. Features that establish outflow condition, the opening pressure (p_{muo}) and the effective size, can be altered separately, leading to distinct forms of obstruction. In normal circumstances, once urethra has assumed its minimal resistance (P_{muo}), there is little further change in detrusor pressure despite increasing flow rate. In *constrictive* obstruction, the opening pressure remains the same but a higher pressure is needed during the mid-voiding. In *compressive* obstruction, the opening pressure is increased because the obstruction acts as the new flow-controlling zone. The pressure is increased not only during mid-voiding but also during initiation and termination of flow. Reproduced from Schäfer W. Principle and clinical application of advanced urodynamic analysis of voiding function. *Urol Clin North Am.* 1990;17:553–6, with permission of Elsevier

whether it is a *compressive* or *constrictive* type of obstruction. The Schäfer nomogram has implemented a "rough linear grading" for the detrusor strength in classes of very weak, weak, normal, and strong. This a simplified qualitative grading scale which is only useful as a guide for clinical judgment when adjustments are made for minimal voided volume. The position of the linPURR is not significantly dependent on the volume voided, but the maximum flow rate (Q_{max}) and the pressure at the maximum flow rate ($P_{detQmax}$) is indeed affected by the degree of bladder distension. It was found that the grading of detrusor strength is less reproducible than outlet function, but can be useful as in the example in Fig. 3, where the patient has the same detrusor strength but improved flow pre- and post-TURP.

ICS (International Continence Society) Nomogram

It was noted that the Abrams-Griffiths nomogram and the Schäfer nomogram had very similar outcomes when classifying men with outlet obstruction. Furthermore, when the Abrams-Griffith nomogram is superimposed on the Schäfer nomogram, the

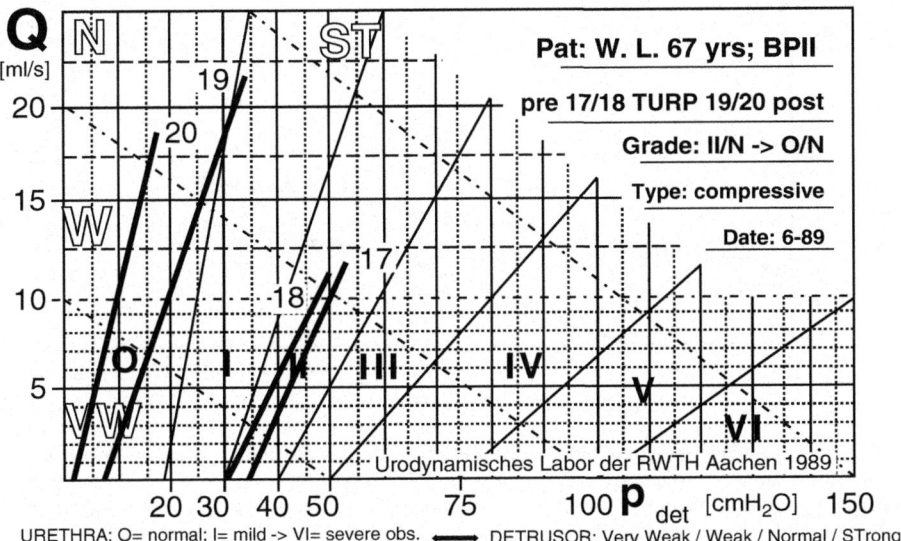

Fig. 4 Schäfer nomogram with a pressure-flow diagram before and after TURP. There are seven zones for grading obstruction (0–VI) and four zones for roughly grading detrusor contraction (Very Weak to Strong). Four voiding studies in a 65-year-old man with typical prostatic symptoms illustrate "mild" obstruction with typical intra-individual variability (*broken lines* in zone I). After transurethral resection, voiding balance is shifted to an optimal normal position (*solid lines* in zone 0). The diagram clearly shows the difference in outflow conditions with essentially unchanged detrusor strength before and after surgery. Each set of curves immediately gives the impression of a rather consistent voiding balance before and after surgery in spite of the significant variability in peak flow of 8–14 and 13–20 ml/s at compatible volumes. Reproduced from Schäfer W. Principle and clinical application of advanced urodynamic analysis of voiding function. *Urol Clin North Am.* 1990;17:553–6, with permission of Elsevier

line separating zone II from zone III on the Schäfer nomogram is equivalent to the line separating obstructed from equivocal on the Abrams-Griffith nomogram (Fig. 4).

The line dividing the obstructed from equivocal was derived by Lim and Abrams in 1995:

$$P_{detQmax} = Y - intercept + 2Q_{max} \qquad (1)$$

The slope of the line is positive 2. The Y-intercept was named to be the Abrams-Griffiths number (AG number), which is 40 cm H_2O at the separation line. **Therefore, points in the obstructed zone will have AG numbers greater than 40, whereas points in the equivocal or unobstructed zones will have AG numbers less than 40. Rearranging the equation to solve for the AG number yielded the following equation:**

$$AG\ Number = P_{detQmax} - 2Q_{max} \qquad (2)$$

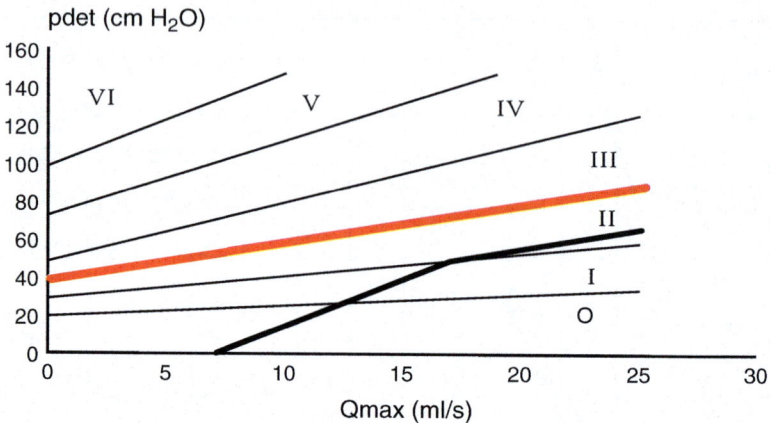

Fig. 5 The Schäfer nomogram superimposed on the Abrams-Griffith nomogram. The *red line* separating obstructed from equivocal on the Abrams-Griffith nomogram is the same as the line separating zone II from zone III on the Schäfer nomogram. Reproduced from Lim CS and Abrams P. The Abrams-Griffith nomogram. *World J Urol*. 1995;13:35, with permission of Springer

Using the combined information from both nomograms, it was concluded that most patients with AG numbers less than 15 are unobstructed, whereas, those with AG numbers 15–40 are equivocal, and those with AG numbers greater than 40 are considered obstructed.

The ICS (International Continence Society) made provisional recommendations regarding both nomograms in 1997 [5]. It was decided that, since the Abrams-Griffiths nomogram is simpler but just as accurate as the Schäfer nomogram in determining obstruction, they would combine both nomograms and adopt an output similar to the Abrams-Griffiths nomogram—obstructed, equivocal, unobstructed. **The AG number was renamed as the***Bladder Outlet Obstruction Index (BOOI)* **. These changes served as the foundation of the ICS nomogram. The cut off values were established: BOOI less than 20 is unobstructed, BOOI between 20 and 40 is considered equivocal, and BOOI greater than 40 is considered obstructed** (Fig. 5). The equivocal zone of the provisional method is similar but not identical to those of the Abrams-Griffiths and linPURR zone II. Slope of the pressure-flow curve can be used to help distinguish those within the equivocal zone.

Bladder Outlet Obstruction in Women: Blaivas-Groutz Nomogram

Bladder outlet obstruction in women has traditionally been difficult to diagnose because the physiology of voiding is different from that in men. The normal pressure generated within the bladder by detrusor muscles is significantly lower in women than in men. As such there has been a lack of standard diagnostic definitions or nomograms, and the prevalence of bladder outlet obstruction in women is not well known but likely to be underestimated [6].

In 2000, Jerry Blaivas, a pioneer in the field of neuro-urology and urodynamics in New York, together with prominent Israeli urogynecologist Asnat Groutz, developed a nomogram based on a urodynamics database of 600 consecutive women referred for evaluation of lower urinary tract symptoms. All 600 women underwent clinical, urodynamic, and radiographic studies. Using several specific and strict inclusion criteria, 50 (8.3 %) women were identified as having bladder outlet obstruction. They matched the obstructed subjects with 50 patients who were confirmed to be unobstructed by patient characteristics, non-invasive uroflow measurements, and pressure-flow studies. The major etiologies of bladder outlet obstruction in women included previous anti-incontinence surgery (20 %), severe genital prolapse (16 %), urethral stricture or narrowing (18 %), and idiopathic (22 %). Other more uncommon etiologies included primary bladder neck obstruction (6 %), urethral diverticulum (6 %), learned voiding dysfunction (4 %), and detrusor-external sphincter dyssynergia (4 %).

Bladder outlet obstruction was defined by one or more of the following inclusion criteria:

1) Free maximum flow rate ≤ 12 ml/s in repeated free-flow studies, combined with a sustained detrusor contraction and $P_{detQmax} \geq 20$ cm H_2O in the pressure-flow study.
2) Obvious radiographic evidence of bladder outlet obstruction in the presence of a sustained detrusor contraction of at least 20 cm H_2O and a poor Q_{max}, regardless of free maximum flow rate.
3) Inability to void with the transurethral catheter in place despite a sustained detrusor contraction of at least 20 cm H_2O.

From the cohort data on these women, a bladder outlet obstruction nomogram was generated using $P_{detQmax}$ and maximum flow rate during unintubated uroflow (freeQmax) (Fig. 6). It is of note that the authors decided to use maximum flow rate based on uroflow without a catheter and not from the pressure-flow study. It has been shown that urodynamic studies using transurethral catheters in women can decrease the flow and falsely elevate the rate of diagnosis of urethral obstruction [7]. The authors also concluded that there was no significant difference between detrusor pressure at maximum flow vs. the overall maximum detrusor pressure during the study; therefore, to simplify the interpretation, it was decided to use the maximum detrusor pressure during any phase of the voiding as the other parameter.

Three major clusters of free $Q_{max}/P_{detQmax}$ plots were identified: 1) low pressure and high flow, 2) high pressure and low flow, 3) low to intermediate pressure and variable flow values. This last group was further divided into two groups, one with mostly obstructed but some clinically unobstructed patients according to the inclusion criteria, and another in which all patients were previously classified as clinically obstructed. These four clusters are the basis for the Blaivas and Groutz nomogram.

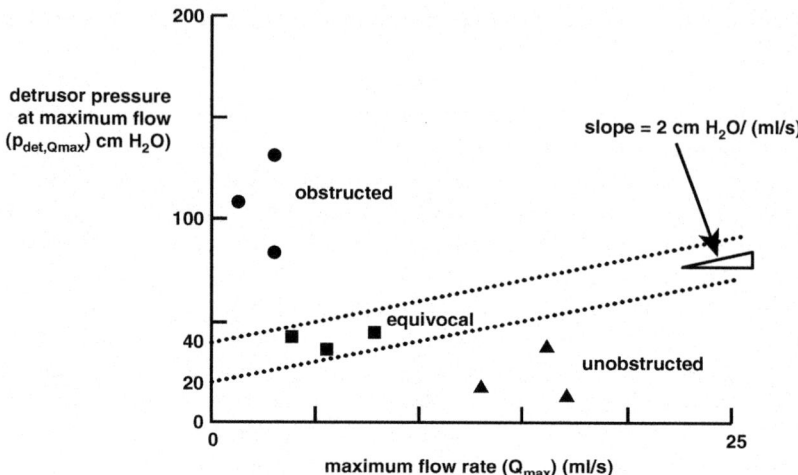

Fig. 6 The International Continence Society (ICS) nomogram. Bladder outlet obstruction index (BOOI) is the value calculated by $P_{detQmax} - 2(Q_{max})$. BOOI less than 20 is unobstructed, BOOI between 20 and 40 is equivocal, BOOI greater than 40 is obstructed. The *points* represent schematically the values of maximum flow rates and detrusor pressure at maximum flow for nine different voids, three in each class. Reproduced from Griffiths D, Hofner K, van Magstrigt R, et al. Standardization of terminology of lower urinary tract function: pressure-flow studies of voiding, urethral resistance and urethral obstruction. *NeurourolUrodyn* 1997;16:1–18, with permission of Wiley

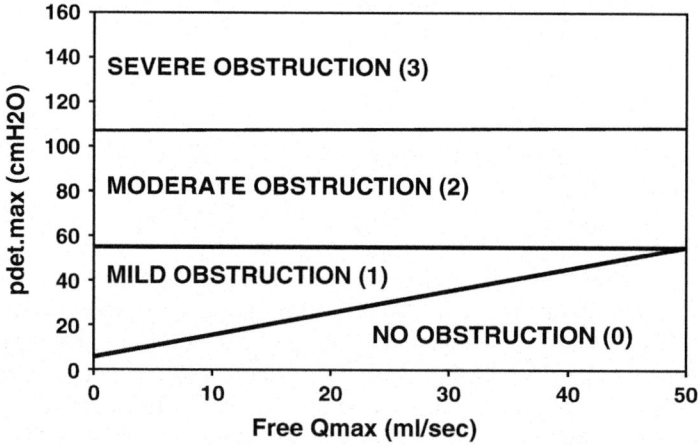

Fig. 7 The Blaivas-Groutz nomogram. Nomogram to aid in the diagnosis of bladder outlet obstruction in women. The nomogram receives a pair of parameters from maximum detrusor pressure during voiding ($P_{detQmax}$) and maximum flow rate during uroflow (free Q_{max}). Patients are classified into four zones; Zone 0: unobstructed, Zone 1: mildly obstructed, Zone 2: moderately obstructed, Zone 3: severely obstructed. Reproduced from Blaivas JG and Groutz A. Bladder outlet obstruction nomogram for women with lower urinary tract symptomatology. *Neurourology and Urodynamics*. 2000;19:553–564, with permission of Wiley

The nomogram is divided into four zones for accurate diagnosis and grading of obstruction: No obstruction in zone 0, mild obstruction in zone I, moderate obstruction in zone II, and severe obstruction in zone III. The boundaries between the four zones are defined as follows: Between unobstructed and mild obstructed: a line with slope 1.0 and intercept 7 cm H_2O. Between mild and moderate obstruction: a horizontal line at $P_{detQmax}$ of 57 cm H_2O. Between moderately and severely obstructed: a horizontal line at $P_{detQmax}$ of 107 cm H_2O.

The nomogram generated by Blaivas and Groutz, is a useful tool to aid in the proper identification of bladder outlet obstruction in women. A recent study using the Blaivas-Groutz nomogram in women with urinary incontinence found that the nomogram might over-diagnose obstruction in this patient group [8]. In their study, Massolt et al. studied 199 women with complaints of urinary incontinence. They underwent multichannel urodynamics testing, free uroflowmetry and were asked to complete the urogenital distress inventory questionnaire. The authors did not find a correlation between the urogenital distress inventory items assessed from the questionnaire and the degree of obstruction as determined by the Blaivas-Groutz nomogram. The authors concluded that the Blaivas-Groutz nomogram gave an unlikely high prevalence of obstruction compared to symptom severity on the urogenital distress inventory.

References

1. Abrams P, Griffiths DJ. The assessment of prostatic obstruction from urodynamic measurement and from residual urine. Br J Urol. 1979;51:129–34.
2. Jensen KM, Jorgensen JB, Mogensen P. Urodynamics in prostatism. II. Prognostic value of pressure-flow study combined with stop-flow test. Scand J Urol Nephrol Suppl. 1988;114:72–7.
3. Rollema HJ, Magstrigt RV. Improved indication and follow-up in transurethral resection of the prostate using the computer program CLIM: a prospective study. J Urol. 1992;148:111–6.
4. Schäfer W. Principle and clinical application of advanced urodynamic analysis of voiding function. Urol Clin North Am. 1990;17:553–6.
5. Griffiths D, Hofner K, van Magstrigt R, et al. Standardization of terminology of lower urinary tract function: pressure-flow studies of voiding, urethral resistance and urethral obstruction. NeurourolUrodyn. 1997;16:1–18.
6. Blaivas JG, Groutz A. Bladder outlet obstruction nomogram for women with lower urinary tract symptomatology. NeurourolUrodyn. 2000;19:553–64.
7. Groutz A, Blaivas JG, Sassone AM. Detrusor pressure-uroflow studies in women: the effect of a 7F transurethral catheter. J Urol. 2000;164:109–40.
8. Massolt ET, Groen J, Vierhout ME. Application of the Blaivas-Groutz outlet obstruction nomogram in women with urinary incontinence. NeurourolUrodyn. 2005;24:237–42.

Ambulatory Urodynamics

Paholo G. Barboglio Romo and E. Ann Gormley

Introduction

Urodynamics remain the gold standard to investigate lower urinary tract symptoms. However, standard urodynamic (SU) testing has significant limitations due to the artificial atmosphere at the time of testing. **Micturition is generally a private experience in most cultural environments whereas most urodynamic testing is seldom private due to the presence of the health care staff performing the test and ideally the physician who will be interpreting the test. Despite the best efforts of the staff in a urodynamic suite to make patients comfortable patients often report embarrassment, anxiety and discomfort during testing.** The patient's position during testing, the presence of catheters, a non-physiologic fill rate, the temperatures of the room and filling solution are all important factors that can either fail to reproduce the patient's urinary symptoms or cause urodynamic findings that do not correlate to the patient's symptoms. Ambulatory urodynamic monitoring (AUM) may be used to mitigate many of these issues.

P.G.B. Romo, M.D., M.P.H.
Section of Urology, Department of Surgery, Dartmouth-Hitchcock Medical Center, 1 Medical Center Drive, Suite # 5B, Lebanon, NH 03756, USA
e-mail: pbarboglio@hitchcock.org

E.A. Gormley, M.D. (✉)
Section of Urology, Department of Surgery, Dartmouth-Hitchcock Medical Center, Mary Hitchcock Hospital, 1 Medical Center Drive, Lebanon, NH 03756, USA
e-mail: Elizabeth.ann.gormley@hitchcock.org

Definition

The International Continence Society (ICS) standardization committee defines ambulatory urodynamic monitoring (AUM) as "any functional test of the lower urinary tract predominantly utilizing natural filling of the urinary tract and reproducing subject's normal activity" [1]. Ambulatory implies that the monitoring is performed outside the urodynamic lab in an attempt to reproduce a more natural, physiologic event in a private environment. The test relies on basic urodynamic principles according to the ICS standardized definitions. Theoretical advantages, in addition to physiologic bladder filling also include a longer duration of testing and more dynamic testing of bladder function in a less artificial environment when compared to standard urodynamics (SU) [1].

Standard and Ambulatory Urodynamics Differences

The major differences between the two techniques are outlined in Table 1. These differences include the environment, the length of the test, the patient's position during testing, the types of catheters used and the fill rate. In both AUM and SU patients must be cooperative and capable of providing feedback regarding their lower urinary symptoms.

Indications

Urodynamic evaluation of a symptomatic patient should be individualized with the goal of investigating a specific urinary problem. Urodynamic testing should be performed to confirm a clinical diagnosis, to potentially alter the management of a

Table 1 Characteristics of SU and AUM

Characteristics	Standard urodynamics (SU)	Ambulatory urodynamic monitoring (AUM)
Environment	Lab with limited privacy	Outside of a lab with less privacy issues
Test length	30–90 min	3–24 h
Patient position	Variable but static. Position, depends on urodynamic equipment and if fluoroscopy is used	Patient moves normally throughout the testing period
Catheters	Catheters attach directly to urodynamic hardware	Catheters have micro-tip transducers that are either attached to, or communicate to a remote device that is attached to the patient
Fill rate	Artificial	Physiologic
Feedback	Patient ideally must be able to verbally describe symptoms	Patient must be capable of indicating symptomatic events

Table 2 ICS indications for ambulatory urodynamics

Failure to reproduce or explain patient's urinary lower urinary symptoms (i.e. patient describes urgency or stress incontinence that is not demonstrated on SU)
Unable to perform SU
Neurogenic bladder
Evaluate outcomes of therapeutic interventions

specific problem or to prevent injury to the upper urinary tracts. Urodynamics is also used to investigate outcomes of therapeutic interventions [2].

AUM has a minimal role in the initial urodynamic evaluation of most patients. They are advantageous when the findings during SU are inconclusive [3]. The ICS recognizes four indications to perform AUM (Table 2) [1].

Ambulatory Urodynamic Monitoring

Historically AUM was performed with standard catheters with intravesical and intra-abdominal pressures measured using fluid filled lines. These lines limited patient mobility. Catheter mounted micro-tip transducers can be used which allow for better patient mobility during AUM. These are secured in the bladder and rectum or vagina with adhesive tape, suture fixation or purpose designed silicone-fixation devices. There are different companies that manufacture portable microprocessors that receive data from the micro-tip transducers. In the last decade wireless Bluetooth® technology has been adopted by some of these companies to avoid the number of wires and simplify the procedure.

Remote devices also have the capacity to allow event marking and recording of urinary symptoms which can be used to perform a digital voiding diary. Leakage events can also be recorded by electronic pads. Data points can be made available via the internet by many of the companies that manufacture these devices. The majority of results can be read or printed from a personal computer making the process very easy for the patient and the physician. The major limitations of AUM are the amount of data produced and the lack of standardization of interpretation and analysis of the data that is conducted by specific software.

Methodology

A detailed explanation is provided to the patient before the test. Instructions to record all urinary symptoms and events, as well as to identify hardware misplacement or malfunction are essential. When using a micro-tip transducer all transducers must be "zeroed" at atmospheric pressure before the catheters are inserted. Unlike a water filled pressure catheter which has a fixed reference point relative to the symphysis a micro-tip transducer does not have a fixed point (See chapter "The Cystometrogram"). Micro-tip transducers will record an erroneous change in pressures when in direct contact with the organ wall or when in contact with other solid material such as stool. Furthermore, the pressures recorded are affected by the vertical height between the vesical and abdominal transducers which can result in negative detrusor values when the patient is in a supine position [3].

As with SU, testing calibration is performed before starting data recording. Each pressure channel must be tested and the patient is asked to cough and to perform a Valsalva maneuver in different positions (supine, sitting and standing) to verify signal quality. Precise positioning and secure fixation are essential to maintain signal quality. The orientation of the transducer should be documented. Transducers should be readjusted if necessary and periodic quality checks should be performed to assess the signal and the patient data input of symptoms and events. It is recommended to have the patient cough or do a Valsalva at regular intervals during the monitoring. This allows for monitoring of signal quality throughout the test which is helpful in the interpretation of the data during the final analysis.

Prior to starting an AUM study a urinary tract infection is ruled out. The catheters are inserted into an empty bladder and ideally an empty rectum. The patient is then asked to get dressed, ambulate, eat, drink and go to the toilet normally at his/her own convenience. When shorter duration studies, 3–4 h, are used some investigators have used protocols where patients are instructed to consume large volume of fluid intake. Patients are instructed to record all coughs or Valsalva maneuvers, any symptoms of urgency and any leakage event in a voiding diary or digitalized into a recording device by pressing a button.

The ICS recommends that an AUM be continued until at least two voiding occasions have been recorded. Additional urodynamics parameters include recording of initiation of voluntary voids, cessation of voluntary voids, episodes of urgency, episodes of discomfort or pain, provocative maneuvers, time and volume of fluid intake, time and volume of urinary leakage and time of pad change [1]. These data points allow for identification of filling versus voiding phase abnormalities.

There are controversies regarding the timing of analyzing the data which is processed through the specific software. Simultaneous recording of urinary symptoms is essential to interpret the results. There can be error and misinterpretation due to the different changes in pressure including pressure changes in the bladder that are volume related. It has been previously described that a second additional transducer can reduce this artifact; however a second transducer can also introduce more confounders simply by adding more data into the analysis and it increases catheter stiffness which may cause alteration of urethral anatomy [4].

Overactive Bladder Syndrome

Ambulatory urodynamics has the advantage of being more sensitive in diagnosing detrusor overactivity (DO) than standard urodynamics (SU) therefore possibly affording an advantage in this patient population. Reports on natural filling cystometry to identify detrusor overactivity (DO), then termed detrusor instability (DI), date back to the late 1970s [5]. In 1980, Thuroff et al. compared AUM to SU and reported a higher sensitivity (60 %) with AUM in comparison to SD (20 %) when studying 10 symptomatic males [6]. Further retrospective studies in the 1990s confirmed the very high sensitivity of AUM to diagnose DI [1, 7]. During this time period the presence of objective DI was a relative contraindication to perform stress incontinence surgery in women with symptoms of stress incontinence and for this reason, urodynamics had a crucial role in the evaluation of urinary incontinence. In 1983 James published on the importance and significance of AUM to reproduce patient urinary symptoms outside the urodynamic suite. Urinary frequency and urgency could be better captured in a less artificial environment with the aim of looking for DI [8].

A prospective study by Webb et al. found a DI rate of 60 % during AUM in 52 women who despite having urinary urgency did not have DI on two prior SU studies [9]. Another study by Vereecken diagnosed DI in 53 % of 100 symptomatic patients with prior negative SU studies [10].

A major criticism of AU is that it may be too sensitive at detecting DO in patients in whom it may not be clinically significant therefore leading to overdiagnosis. There is no question that AU is highly sensitive to diagnose DO in symptomatic patients. However a prospective study by Salvatore et al. on 26 asymptomatic women (mean age 32 years) showed an abnormally high finding of DO in 17 patients (65 %) which was reduced to 3 patients (11.5 %) when two urethral transducers and a voiding diary were used. In this study AUM testing was carried out for up to 4 h [11]. It is unclear how the investigators analyzed all increases in detrusor amplitude associated with symptoms or leakage using two transducers. There was also a lack of blinding which may have led to investigator bias. Although the authors recommended a number of strategies to help decrease the potential for over diagnosis, these findings have never been reproduced in a larger trial.

There is one RCT by Radley et al. on 106 symptomatic patients who were subjected to both SU and AUM in a random order. DO was detected in 32 and 70 tests of video SU and AUM ($p<0.001$) respectively. DO associated with urge incontinence was noted in 39 AUM studies of which half of these patients had a negative SU. Patient's questionnaires were correlated to urodynamic findings and 85 % women believed that their symptoms were reproduced by AUM vs 66.7 % during SU ($p=0.013$). The authors concluded that conventional studies should be interpreted with caution since AUM diagnosed a higher rate of DO in symptomatic women which highly correlated to patient's OAB symptoms and Quality of Life questionnaires. Interestingly there were four women with DO on SU with a prior negative AUM study [12].

Stress Incontinence

There is limited data supporting the utility of AUM to diagnose urodynamic stress urinary incontinence (SUI). Bo et al. reported an increased sensitivity for detecting SUI when AUM was performed for 45 min during physical activity in comparison to SU [13]. A RCT by Radley et al. showed no significant difference between AUM and SU when assessing SUI in 106 symptomatic patients. There were 42 women diagnosed with SUI on SU versus 34 on AUM (p=0.629) [12].

In the Webb study that was discussed earlier, in addition to finding that AUM was more sensitive in the detection of DI in 52 women, urodynamic SUI was found in 10 (19 %) women during AUM of which three (3/10) had both urodynamic SUI and DI. In this study the authors commented on the importance of AUM in symptomatic patients with mixed urinary incontinence when assessing for DI with prior unremarkable SU [9].

Today, the utility of urodynamics in the diagnosis of SUI is being questioned. The AUA's Guidelines on the surgical treatment of stress incontinence state that as a standard, the evaluation of the index patient should include "a focused history, a focused physical examination, objective demonstration of SUI, assessment of post void residual and a urinalysis. Additional diagnostic tests should be performed to assess the integrity and function of the lower urinary tract if one is unable to make a definitive diagnosis based on the initial evaluation, if there are concomitant overactive bladder symptoms, or other findings that make the diagnosis of SUI questionable" [14]. Although other testing, including urodynamic testing is advocated for the patient with concomitant overactive bladder symptoms in the AUA Stress incontinence guidelines, the AUA Urodynamic Guidelines specify that in the patient with mixed incontinence "the absence of DO on a single urodynamic study does not exclude it as a causative agent for their symptoms. Therefore, urodynamic findings should be interpreted in the context of the global assessment, including examination, diaries and residual urine as well as other pertinent information" [15].

AUM testing has played an important role in diagnosing DO in patients with mixed incontinence or other complex genitourinary histories, particularly in the patient with an unremarkable SU. Through the use of AUM we now know that some patients with symptoms of urgency who may not have DO on a SU test may have it on AUM. If a patient with SUI reports urge symptoms regardless if they do or do not have DO on SU she should be counseled that a surgical intervention to manage her SUI may not address her urgency symptoms and these urgency symptoms may improve, stay the same or increase in severity after surgery. Given the increased sensitivity of AUM to diagnose DO, AUM could play an important role in assessing for DO in the patient with mixed incontinence and a complex genitourinary history with an unremarkable SU.

Bladder Outlet Obstruction

Urodynamic testing is considered an optional test in the American Urologic Association (AUA) Guidelines for Benign Prostatic Hyperplasia. SU should be performed to determine the presence of obstruction when invasive and, or irreversible treatments are considered and if the outcome of a pressure flow test might impact the choice of the intervention [16]. The diagnosis of bladder outlet obstruction is made with urodynamics and relies on a linear relation between detrusor pressure and urinary flow at the time of volitional voiding. Obstruction is diagnosed when there is a high detrusor pressure with low flow (See chapter "The Pressure Flow Study"). Detrusor pressure and urinary flow can be plotted on the Abrams-Griffiths or Schafer nomograms to diagnose obstruction (See chapter "Nomograms"). The role of AUM in the setting of BOO is limited. As previously stated AUM studies are more likely to detect DO, but this does not predict outcome following surgery to relief bladder outlet obstruction. Voiding pressures have been shown to be higher during AUM, but this has proven not to impact final diagnosis based on nomogram data [17].

Neurogenic Bladder

The AUA Urodynamic Guidelines recommends urodynamics during the initial evaluation of patients with relevant neurologic conditions with or without symptoms and when appropriate, as part of ongoing follow-up [15]. **The purpose of a urodynamic investigation in a patient with a neurogenic bladder is to assess the bladder pressure during filling and voiding and to assess the outlet during these two stages. However, the role of AUM in neurogenic bladder has been studied primarily in spinal cord injury patients and its role is still controversial.**

AUM could potentially be used in the neurogenic patient population given the mobility limitations and the difficulties that can exist in measuring incontinence episodes. Natural filling by AUM could provide better understanding of the true bladder capacity and bladder pressure in this patient population.

Martens et al. performed a prospective study that confirmed a higher sensitivity of AUM to diagnose DO, but the authors emphasized that this had no impact on the patients' outcomes. They concluded that there was no role for AUM in the standard primary urodynamic workup in spinal cord injury cases when SU are performed appropriately [18].

Kim et al. also found more DO when using AUM with a personal device assistant for data collection. The AUM device they used utilized EMG patches to calculate abdominal pressure which was shown to have excellent correlation to rectal pressure. They studied 28 patients with spinal cord injury and compared their new device to SU. The authors found that neurogenic DO was more common with AUM in patients with areflexic bladders. They also found that neurogenic DO leading to incontinence occurred at lower volumes when using AUM. In this study patients were not filled at a physiologic rate since they were asked to drink 500 ml of water and were given 10 mg of IV furosemide with the aim being to reduce the amount of time that the study took. Other limitations of this study were that AUM was performed 2 h after SU and most studies were performed in a hospital bed and not in an ambulatory manner [19].

Virseda et al., studied 64 consecutive patients with stable spinal cord injuries who underwent SU and AUM 24 h apart and found significant correlation coefficient when assessing bladder capacity (0.74), maximum detrusor pressure at involuntary contraction (0.84) and post void residual (0.74). However they found no significant correlation when assessing end filling detrusor pressure [20].

These findings support the use of AUM in the neurogenic patient if for some reason SU cannot be performed or if SU are performed and are inconclusive. As with DO in the non-neurogenic patient AUM detects more DO in the neurogenic patient.

Future Technology

The ideal urodynamic system would consist of a minimally invasive catheter-less device that would allow long term monitoring of bladder pressure without artifact. New devices have been created to measure intravesical pressure. Wille et al. have created an intravesical device to measure pressure, a hand held device and an alarm pad which allows for the performance of a long term urodynamic study without a catheter. The authors designed a silicone coated C-shaped flexible capsule that can be elongated to allow insertion by cystoscopy. Following insertion the device will then regain its original C-configuration to avoid ejection during micturition [21].

This innovative device is still been tested for safety purposes. To date in vitro investigations of the capsule and battery showed no device-related toxicity. The capsule can function up to 3 days or more to measure urodynamic parameters, patient's urinary symptoms can be recorded through the hand held device and urinary leakage is identified by the alarm pad in a simultaneous fashion [21].

We believe that a catheter-less device that can measure urodynamic parameters could replace and re-invent the concept of AUM. Although this minimally invasive system may allow a more accurate understanding of the bladder function, there are still many questions to be answered.

Conclusion

Ambulatory urodynamics have not proven to impact patient's outcomes when compared to standard urodynamics. There may be a role for AUM in those patients where a complete evaluation with voiding diaries and validated questionnaires and standard urodynamics is still inconclusive. New technologies using catheter free devices are likely to improve ambulatory urodynamics.

References

1. van Waalwijk van Doorn E, Anders K, Khullar V, Kulseng-Hanssen S, Pesce F, Robertson A, Rosario D, Schafer W. Standardization of ambulatory urodynamic monitoring: report of the Standardization Sub-Committee of the International Continence Society for Ambulatory Urodynamic Studies. NeurourolUrodyn. 2000;19(2):113–25.
2. Gammie A, Clarkson B, Constantinou C, Damaser M, Drinnan M, Geleijnse G, Griffiths D, Rosier P, Schafer W, Van Mastrigt R, International Continence Society Urodynamic Equipment Working Group. International Continence Society guidelines on urodynamic equipment performance. NeurourolUrodyn. 2014;33(4):370–9.
3. Abrams P, Andersson KE, Birder L, Brubaker L, Cardozo L, Chapple C, Cottenden A, Davila W, de Ridder D, Dmochowski R, Drake M, Dubeau C, Fry C, Hanno P, Smith JH, Herschorn S, Hosker G, Kelleher C, Koelbl H, Khoury S, Madoff R, Milsom I, Moore K, Newman D, Nitti V, Norton C, Nygaard I, Payne C, Smith A, Staskin D, Tekgul S, Thuroff J, Tubaro A, Vodusek D, Wein A, Wyndaele JJ, Members of Committees & Fourth International Consultation on Incontinence. Fourth International Consultation on Incontinence Recommendations of the International Scientific Committee: Evaluation and treatment of urinary incontinence, pelvic organ prolapse, and fecal incontinence. NeurourolUrodyn. 2010;29(1):213–40.
4. van Waalwijk van Doorn ES, Meier AM, Ambergen AW, Janknegt RA. Ambulatory urodynamics: extramural testing of the lower and upper urinary tract by Holter monitoring of cystometrogram, uroflowmetry, and renal pelvic pressures. Urol Clin North Am. 1996;23(3):345–71.
5. Abrams P, Blaivas JG, Stanton SL, Andersen JT. The standardisation of terminology of lower urinary tract function. The International Continence Society Committee on Standardisation of Terminology. Scand J Urol Nephrol Suppl. 1988;114:5–19.
6. Thuroff JW, Jonas U, Frohneberg D, Petri E, Hohenfellner R. Telemetric urodynamic investigations in normal males. Urol Int. 1980;35(6):427–34.
7. Heslington K, Hilton P. Ambulatory monitoring and conventional cystometry in asymptomatic female volunteers. Br J Obstet Gynaecol. 1996;103(5):434–41.
8. James ED. The bladder during physical activity: further views on natural-filling urodynamic investigations. Br J Urol. 1983;55(5):570.
9. Webb RJ, Ramsden PD, Neal DE. Ambulatory monitoring and electronic measurement of urinary leakage in the diagnosis of detrusor instability and incontinence. Br J Urol. 1991;68(2):148–52.
10. Vereecken RL, van Nuland T. Detrusor pressure in ambulatory versus standard urodynamics. NeurourolUrodyn. 1998;17(2):129–33.
11. Salvatore S, Khullar V, Cardozo L, Anders K, Zocchi G, Soligo M. Evaluating ambulatory urodynamics: a prospective study in asymptomatic women. BJOG. 2001;108(1):107–11.
12. Radley SC, Rosario DJ, Chapple CR, Farkas AG. Conventional and ambulatory urodynamic findings in women with symptoms suggestive of bladder overactivity. J Urol. 2001;166(6):2253–8.
13. Bo K, Stien R, Kulseng-Hanssen S, Kristofferson M. Clinical and urodynamic assessment of nulliparous young women with and without stress incontinence symptoms: a case-control study. Obstet Gynecol. 1994;84(6):1028–32.
14. Dmochowski RR, Blaivas JM, Gormley EA, Juma S, Karram MM, Lightner DJ, Luber KM, Rovner ES, Staskin DR, Winters JC, Appell RA, Whetter LE, Female Stress Urinary Incontinence Update Panel of the American Urological Association Education and Research, Inc. Update of AUA guideline on the surgical management of female stress urinary incontinence. J Urol. 2010;183(5):1906–14.
15. Winters JC, Dmochowski RR, Goldman HB, Herndon CD, Kobashi KC, Kraus SR, Lemack GE, Nitti VW, Rovner ES, Wein AJ, American Urological Association & Society of Urodynamics, Female Pelvic Medicine & Urogenital Reconstruction. Urodynamic studies in adults: AUA/SUFU guideline. J Urol. 2012;188(6 Suppl):2464–72.

16. McVary KT, Roehrborn CG, Avins AL, Barry MJ, Bruskewitz RC, Donnell RF, Foster Jr HE, Gonzalez CM, Kaplan SA, Penson DF, Ulchaker JC, Wei JT. Update on AUA guideline on the management of benign prostatic hyperplasia. J Urol. 2011;185(5):1793–803.
17. Robertson AS, Griffiths C, Neal DE. Conventional urodynamics and ambulatory monitoring in the definition and management of bladder outflow obstruction. J Urol. 1996;155(2):506–11.
18. Martens FM, van Kuppevelt HJ, Beekman JA, Heijnen IC, D'Hauwers KW, Heesakkers JP. No primary role of ambulatory urodynamics for the management of spinal cord injury patients compared to conventional urodynamics. NeurourolUrodyn. 2010;29(8):1380–6.
19. Kim KS, Song CG. Availability of a newly devised ambulatory urodynamics monitoring system based on personal device assistance in patients with spinal cord injury. Comput Methods Programs Biomed. 2012;106(3):260–73.
20. Virseda M, Salinas J, Esteban M, Mendez S. Reliability of ambulatory urodynamics in patients with spinal cord injuries. NeurourolUrodyn. 2013;32(4):387–92.
21. Wille S, Tenholte D, Engelmann U. A system for long-term urodynamic studies without catheters. Eur Urol. 2013;63(5):966–8.

Bedside Urodynamics

Andrew C. Peterson

Introduction

Rehfish first described the study of the lower urinary tract in 1897 with specific instruments devised to measure mictuuration [1]. Over the next century there were significant advancements in this field leading to the development of the cystometrograph in 1927 as an early urodynamic instruments for measuring bladder pressure during storage and voiding [2]. This was followed by the invention of the urine flowmeter by Drake in 1948 [3]. In the 1950s Hinman and Miller pioneered the development of simultaneous radiographic imaging done in conjunction with the bladder pressure studies [4]. **The term urodynamics was finally coined by Davis in 1953 to denote the study of the storage and emptying phases of the urinary bladder.** As one can see, initially urodynamics consisted of very simple "bedside" tests with the examiner simply observing the act of voiding and the strength of the stream in order to comment on the function of the bladder [5].

As we have discussed throughout this book, complex urodynamics are becoming increasingly available, standardized and easy to use. Excellent outlines and guidelines have been established to make the studies consistent among different facilities and easier to conduct [6]. However, there still remains debate as to when these complex, expensive and invasive tests are to be performed. **Bedside urodynamics refers to testing that may be performed without the use of machines, invasive monitors and expensive equipment** [7]. These can be extremely useful when combined with other factors used to evaluate the patient with voiding dysfunction such as; the history and physical examination, urination diary, pad weight test, and

---

A.C. Peterson, M.D. (✉)
Department of Surgery, Division of Urology, Duke University Medical Center,
1113 Davison Building, DUMC, Durham, NC 27710, USA
e-mail: drew.peterson@duke.edu

© Springer International Publishing Switzerland 2016
A.C. Peterson, M.O. Fraser (eds.), *Practical Urodynamics for the Clinician*,
DOI 10.1007/978-3-319-20834-3_12

laboratory evaluations. This technique of evaluation for these patients should not be underestimated because they may often yield key information that may help to characterize the problem more clearly leading to a plethora of information on the etiology of incontinence and voiding dysfunction [8]. **Bedside urodynamics are less expensive, less invasive, and less complex to perform and utilize no specialized equipment or techniques.** As we will see, many of the components of urodynamics discussed in the book up to this point may be classified as noninvasive bedside urodynamics (urination diary, pad weight test, post void residual, uroflow test). Similar to invasive complex urodynamics these tests should always be performed starting from the simplest and least invasive while progressing to the more comprehensive examination when indicated. Also, as mentioned previously in other chapters not all components of the bedside urodynamics will be required in every case as the clinician must be reminded to continuously tailor the examination to the clinical scenario.

Patient Selection

The 2002 international continence Society (good urodynamic practices) report clearly recommends basic requirements for the conduct of urodynamics including the utilization of a comprehensive history, physical exam, the use of a voiding diary, and a stress test with objective demonstration of the incontinence [6]. When the clinician wishes to obtain more data on the voiding dysfunction, bedside urodynamics provides the opportunity to do just this. **Not all patients are good candidates for bedside urodynamics. The best candidates for this simple testing are those who have no prior incontinence surgery,havesimple/straightforward clinical questions and clear symptoms of stress incontinence, urge with urge incontinence, or bladder overactivity** [7].

The Instruments Used in Bedside Urodynamics

As we see in the other chapters in this textbook, the instruments that are utilized for simplified bedside urodynamic testing should be of no surprise. These include the voiding diary, post void residual, uroflow, and bedside cystometry. Each of these tools will be discussed in detail as they pertain to bedside urodynamics without the need to repeat and expand upon discussions already presented elsewhere. Regardless of whether they are complex urodynamics or bedside urodynamics it is important to continuously strive to optimize the quality of any of these studies in order to increase the possibility of gaining usable information. **One of the basic tenants of any urodynamics (bedside urodynamics or the complex fluorourodynamics with video) is the prospective evaluation of a clinical question with specific** relation to the patient's complaint [9]. **Therefore, all of these studies should always be conducted with constant and consistent patient interaction between the clinician and the subject.** This interaction should include discussion on the patient's symptoms and whether they are being replicated within the artificial environment of the study.

Uroflow

Uroflowmetry is noninvasive, inexpensive and invaluable in screening patients with voiding dysfunction [10]. It gives the clinician an estimate and representation of the patient's ability to void with a certain speed and volume over an amount of time. We feel this noninvasive test should precede any other urodynamic studies. It is easy to perform and quickly provides data on both storage and voiding symptoms. These studies should be conducted with as much privacy as possible and the patient should be asked to void when they feel a normal desire. Ideally two or more tests should be performed and the addition of a noninvasive postvoid residual volume measurement by ultrasound adds to the value of the study.

Usually, these measurements are obtained with complex uroflow machines based off of rotating disc inertia, weight and density of the fluid, or capacitance as the fluid fills a colander (See chapter "Noninvasive Urodynamics"). These machines are extremely valuable in everyday clinical evaluation of patients and provide graphic representation and recording of the void. However, much more simple ways of measuring this are available; in many cases a simple container to measure the voided volume and a stopwatch are all that are needed in order to complete these tasks and provide the clinician with a total voided volume and average flow rate.

In order to provide a competent and interpretable flow test, the patient should start out with a full bladder that is not yet uncomfortable, preferably estimating the functional capacity as outlined on the voiding diary. Classically the patient needed to void at least 150 mL in order to make this a valid study. However, if the patient was too full it may over extend in the bladder and result in abnormal results. Therefore, to avoid these pitfalls one should always counsel patient that they should perform a noninvasive uroflow with the similar feelings as to their functional capacity on the voiding diary [11].

The average flow is easily calculated by measuring the voided total volume, measuring the time it takes to void out that total volume and then calculating an average flow by dividing the volume by the voided time:

$$\text{Voided volume}(CC) / \text{voided time}(s) = \text{average flow rate}(CC/s)$$

The average flow rate should be at least 8 cc/s for any adult (which corresponds to a maximum flow rate of 15 cc/s which is considered normal) [11]. To help augment this average flow rate calculation from noninvasive/bedside urodynamics it is important for the patient to give the clinician information on the quality of the urinary stream such as force, whether it was continuous or interrupted, and whether they had to push to void past any obstructive symptoms. These may be extremely valuable when taking everything in the light on a global basis.

Once again it's important to state that the uroflow test is a screening test and true bladder pathology must be evaluated definitively with invasive urodynamics in situations that require the indicated test as discussed elsewhere in this book (See chapter "The Pressure Flow Study"). Interpretation of the uroflow test and the clinical relevance of these findings are discussed elsewhere in the book in the reader is encouraged to visit those chapters for details.

Postvoid Residual

The postvoid residual (PVR) is one of the most widely used noninvasive, noncomplex studies of the bladder and holds great relevance within urology and primary care. The volume that a patient leaves within the bladder after the end of voiding provides a plethora of information about not only the bladder's ability to contract, but may give information on obstruction and incontinence. **The amount of urine left within the bladder after voiding may be measured with two common techniques; ultrasound and bladder catheterization.** Bladder ultrasonography provides a rapid noninvasive method to estimate the amount of urine left. This carries with it a low risk of invasive complications such as infection and injury to the urethra [12]. Disadvantages of this technique as compared to direct measurement with catheterization include the concern about inaccuracy of the volume estimated. The equipment needed to perform ultrasonography may be complex and require special techniques to use. However, with the implementation of ultrasonography across many subspecialty fields including emergency rooms, outpatient clinics and the inpatient care wards this technology is becoming increasingly available. In addition to this, purpose specific scanners are now available commercially that are designed specifically to determine the postvoid residual. These are available for use by clinicians and nurses with minimal training and experience.

In patients with a body habitus that does not lend itself to ultrasonography (morbid obesity), or in situations where the ultrasonography may not be available, straight catheterization with a small catheter (12–14 French red rubber) is perfectly appropriate to determine the PVR. Additionally, when the clinician has decided that a bedside cystometrogram is required, placement of the catheter will be the first step in this task therefore allowing the bladder to drain for an additional minute will enable the clinician to evaluate for the PVR.

Interpretation of the post void residual and the clinical relevance of this is discussed elsewhere in the book and the reader is encouraged to visit those chapters for details (See chapter "Noninvasive Urodynamics").

Cystometry

The more invasive component of bedside urodynamics is the cystometrogram and one would not need to do this study if they've already decided to move forward with invasive multichannel/fluorourodynamics. Therefore the indications for this pertain to those patients with simple straightforward questions. Patients with an unsuccessful prior surgical intervention, those who fail medical therapy or those with a neurologic complaint typically would not be good candidates for the bedside urodynamics as they typically would be scheduled for formal more complex urodynamics [7]. **While the data garnered from a bedside urodynamics cystometrogram are limited, the study may be very helpful in assessing three key components; bladder capacity, sensation and presence of detrusor over activity.** This can be an invaluable study in those patients with straightforward symptoms of stress and urgency incontinence as well as bladder over activity.

The "eyeball" or bedside urodynamics cystogram is performed with only a 60-mL syringe, urethral catheter and sterile water. Because the equipment requirements are minimal for this type of cystometrogram and catheters are readily available this type of testing may be performed quickly and with significant cost savings. Most clinicians can conduct the bedside cystometrogram with small urethral catheters in order to minimize discomfort (12 French). The patient is initially asked to void and the catheter is placed by the clinician. This is allowed to drain for 1–2 min therefore establishing the postvoid residual.

After establishing the postvoid residual the "eyeball" cystometrogram is performed. The catheter is left in place in the bladder and an irrigating syringe is attached with the plunger removed. The bladder is then filled under gravity by placing sterile saline into the Toomey syringe holding the syringe 15 cm above the symphysis pubis (Fig. 1). From this, bladder capacity, sensation, and information about detrusor instability may be obtained. While the filling is performed slowly the patient is asked to give information on sensation, initial desire to void and strong desired to void. The final capacity which would be the total bladder capacity is determined by the patient's reports of being full to the point of discomfort.

Detrusor overactivity and compliance of the bladder may be evaluated subjectively by watching the meniscus of the fluid within the irrigating syringe during filling. If it continuously and smoothly fills the bladder then one can assume there are no uninhibited contractions. However, with detrusor overactivity and uninhibited contractions one may see the meniscus move up and down repeatedly during filling often accompanied by symptoms expressed from the patient. The need to elevate the syringe to maintain filling corresponds to an increase in bladder pressure which may be secondary to bladder contractions, reduced compliance, or abdominal straining.

Capacity and compliance may also be subjectively evaluated with this method. This may manifest as slow bladder filling or in intermittent stoppages of the bladder filling on passive non-invasive bedside urodynamics. Usually, in a normal compliance bladder with low-pressure and good capacity the fluid will continue to fill the

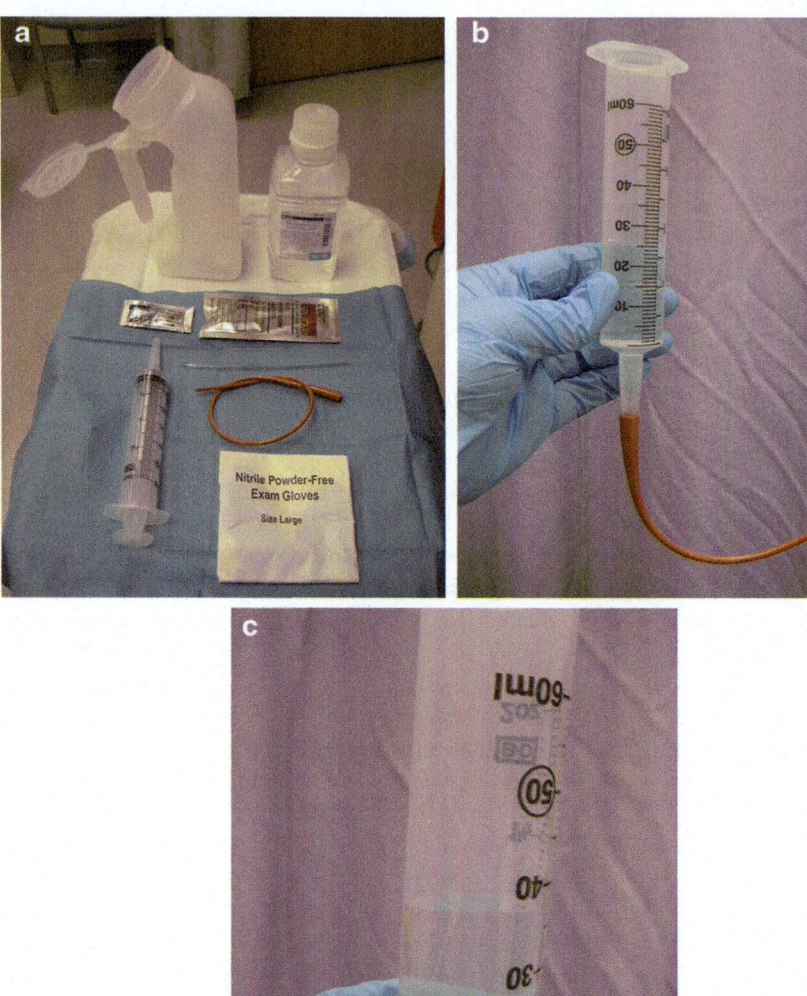

Fig. 1 (**a**) Bedside urodynamics may be conducted with minimal equipment; A small 12 French catheter, irrigating syringe, sterile gloves, lubricant jelly, fluid and a urinal. (**b**) The plunger is removed from the irrigating syringe. This is attached to the small catheter which has been placed into the bladder. It may be held just above the pubic symphysis of the patient who is supine and filled under gravity with room temperature sterile saline. (**c**) The clinician can estimate bladder capacity, compliance and the presence of uninhibited contractions (detrusor overactivity) during filling and storage phase by observing the movement of the meniscus within the irrigating syringe

bladder until the total bladder capacity as determined by that patients urination diary is reached. However, slow bladder filling or intermittent stoppage of the bladder filling may indicate loss of compliance.

The largest drawback of "bedside" urodynamics and this type of cystometrogram is that no estimate of the contractility of thebladdercan be made. Without directly measuring the pressures of the bladder during contractions it is impossible to establish whether contractility is normal and the patient's motor system is intact.

Summary

Bedside urodynamics may provide a significant adjunctive maneuver for the clinician when access to complex urodynamics is neither feasible nor indicated. Despite the low complexity, much data can be garnered with this cost-effective, minimally invasive and simple testing.

References

1. Rehfish E. Ueber den Mechanismus des Harneblasenverschlusses und der Harnentleerung. Virchows Arch Fur Anat U Fur Klin Med. 1897;150:111.
2. Rose D. Determination of bladder pressure with the cystometer. JAMA. 1927;88:151.
3. Drake W. The uroflowmeter: an aid to the study of the lower urinary tract. J Urol. 1948;59:650.
4. Hinman F, Miller G, Nickle A, Miller E. Vesical physiology demonstrated by cineradiography and serial roentgenography. Radiology. 1954;62:713.
5. Davis DM. The hydrodynamics of the upper urinary tract (urodynamics). Ann Surg. 1954;140:839.
6. Schafer W, Abrams P, Liao L, Mattiasson A, Pesce F, Spangberg A, et al. Good urodynamic practices: uroflowmetry, filling cystometry, and pressure-flow studies. Neurourol Urodyn. 2002;21:261.
7. Rayome RG. Simple urodynamic techniques. J Wound Ostomy Continence Nurs. 1995;22:17.
8. Wein AJ, English WS, Whitmore KE. Office urodynamics. Urol Clin North Am. 1988;15:609.
9. Winters JC, Dmochowski RR, Goldman HB, Herndon CD, Kobashi KC, Kraus SR, et al. Urodynamic studies in adults: AUA/SUFU guideline. J Urol. 2012;188:2464.
10. Bray A, Griffiths C, Drinnan M, Pickard R. Methods and value of home uroflowmetry in the assessment of men with lower urinary tract symptoms: a literature review. Neurourol Urodyn. 2012;31:7.
11. Jorgensen JB, Jensen KM. Uroflowmetry. Urol Clin North Am. 1996;23:237.
12. Newman DK, Smith DA. A portable bladder scanner. Nurse Pract Forum. 1991;2:243.

Practical Urodynamics in Children

Sherry S. Ross and John S. Wiener

Introduction

Urodynamic testing is an important tool in the evaluation of children with refractory urinary incontinence or with disorders predisposing to neurogenic or anatomically altered bladders. Its purpose is to determine the physiological variables of filling, storage and emptying of the bladder and their coordination with the sphincteric mechanism. **Urodynamics provides accurate assessment of lower urinary tract function and may identify those children with deleterious bladder pressures which may cause damage to the upper urinary tract.**

Indications

Non-neurogenic Bladder

Children often present for evaluation if they fail to attain continence by normal age of toilet training, which typically should be complete by the fourth birthday. Causes include overactive bladder, dysfunctional voiding, underactive bladder, bladder outlet obstruction or voiding postponement [1] which may be associated with urinary incontinence or other lower urinary tract symptoms such as urgency, frequency, and holding maneuvers. The main goal of urodynamics in this population is to determine if urinary problems are neurological or functional in origin.

In children with no known etiology for abnormal urinary behaviors, urodynamics should be performed only after a thorough evaluation has been conducted and simple treatment measures have failed. Evaluation includes completion of a voiding questionnaire, clinical examination, uroflow with post-void residual (PVR) determination, and ultrasound imaging [2]. Voiding cystourethrogram (VCUG) may be indicated as well, especially in boys to evaluate the urethra for congenital obstructive lesions. Conservative first line treatment such as timed voids, elimination of caffeinated products, and improved toileting habits and posture are recommended. Inquiry into bowel function cannot be emphasized enough, as approximately 50 % of children with lower urinary tract conditions have bowel dysfunction described as constipation or encopresis [3]. Treatment of constipation with over-the-counter stimulants or enemas may improve urinary tract symptoms. In children with severe constipation refractory to medical therapy, referral to a pediatric gastroenterologist may be necessary. The triad of urinary tract infections (UTI), constipation and voiding symptoms such as incontinence, urgency, and frequency has been termed dysfunctional elimination syndrome (DES). These children may benefit from anti-cholinergic medications and up to 80–94 % may benefit from biofeedback to teach pelvic floor relaxation [4, 5]. Children with DES typically have normal sensation, and urodynamics is invasive and can be painful. Furthermore, they often do not understand the utility of urodynamics and may not be a willing participant in the study. **Therefore, urodynamic evaluation should be reserved for those children who fail to respond to conservative therapy. At some point, though, urodynamics should be entertained in children with non-neurologic voiding dysfunction as studies have demonstrated pathological findings that can tailor appropriate therapies based on objective urodynamic findings** [6]. Perhaps more importantly, urodynamics may be a useful adjuvant in the diagnosis of occult neuropathies, such as tethered spinal cord, when physical examination findings are equivocal or the need for neurosurgical intervention is in question [7].

Neurogenic Bladder

Urodynamics is indicated in children with a suspected diagnosis of neurogenic bladder. Children with spinal cord injury, spina bifida, VACTERL (vertebral, anal, cardiac, tracheal, esophageal, renal and limb abnormalities), caudal regression, and sacral agenesis are at high risk for neurogenic bladder and should undergo baseline urodynamic evaluation within the first few months after birth or diagnosis. Up to 57 % of children with anorectal malformations [8] have MRI evidence of spinal abnormalities, and children with cutaneous finding such as hairy patches, deviated gluteal cleft, skin dimple and dermal vascular malformations may have spinal abnormalities that result in neuropathic bladder function.

Urodynamics can both diagnose and characterize pathological aspects of the neurogenic bladder and identify those at high risk of bladder deterioration and renal failure [9]. Early identification of neurogenic bladder can allow implementation of therapies with the goal of a bladder of normal capacity and compliance that stores urine at a low pressure and empties completely. **Unlike adults, children are growing, and bladder physiology can change over time, so urodynamics should be repeated. The optimal schedule for repeating urodynamic evaluation remains elusive. In many patients with neurogenic bladder, urodynamics remains the primary means of determining the efficacy of therapy and need for surgical intervention since altered neurological innervation interferes with clinical symptoms and radiological imaging alone cannot determine bladder dysfunction.**

Preparing for Urodynamic Evaluation in Children

Pre-study Considerations

Urodynamic studies can be intimidating to both parents and children. **To insure that information obtained during urodynamics is accurate and to prevent the need for repeat studies, thorough evaluation and proper planning is important**. Prior to scheduling urodynamics, it is imperative that a complete history and physical examination is performed. Information including prenatal history, birth and development, as well as medical and surgical history are important to understand factors which may influence bladder function. In select children, a voiding and stooling diary which includes fluid intake is important to document habits which may play a role in urinary and stool incontinence. Physical examination should include evaluation of the spine, lower extremities and genitalia. Laboratory studies, including urinalysis and urine culture, are important to rule out UTI, and serum creatinine is helpful to estimate renal function. Renal-bladder ultrasound is useful to exclude upper tract anomalies or injury and allows some evaluation of bladder anatomy and function with bladder wall thickness and measurement of pre- and post-void volumes. VCUG provides anatomical assessment of the bladder and urethra—the latter being more important in boys—and can diagnose vesicoureteral reflux (VUR) which can influence urodynamic parameters such as functional bladder capacity measurements. Alternatively, the need for VCUG can be obviated by videourodynamics with fluoroscopic evaluation of the bladder (and upper tracts, if VUR present), but imaging detail, particularly of the urethra, may be inferior to VCUG.

Considerations of additional factors that may influence bladder function are important when planning urodynamic studies in children. Constipation can significantly affect bladder function. In addition, large stool loads can make rectal catheter placement cumbersome, resulting in catheter placement into stool which alters pressure readings or expulsion of the catheter during the study as well as soiling of EMG patches, if used. Laxatives given 2–3 days before the study or rectal enemas should be considered in constipated patients.

A thorough history of medications that can affect bladder and urethral sphincter function is critical. If possible, medications known to affect bladder and sphincter function should be held prior to the study, or urodynamic studies should be delayed until medication treatment course is complete. Management of medications given specifically for bladder function, such as anticholinergics, depends on the overall goal of the study. For baseline urodynamic evaluation of the neurogenic bladder or in children with non-neurogenic bladder who have been placed on anticholinergic for symptoms, anticholinergic medications should be held for at least 2 days prior to the study, if immediate release, or 7 days if extended release. If anticholinergic therapy was initiated after baseline urodynamics, follow up studies should be repeated in 3–6 months to determine if bladder function has improved. This is especially important in patients with bladder pressures >40 cm H_2O since renal function may be compromised if pressures remain high in spite of medication therapy. For follow up studies, it is important to ensure that the medication was taken on schedule prior to the study.

Children with evidence of UTI, as indicated by symptoms or elevations in urinary WBC on urinalysis, with or without positive urine culture, should not undergo urodynamic evaluation. Resulting bladder inflammation may affect detrusor compliance or cause detrusor overactivity and lead to false results. Furthermore, creating high bladder pressures during filling in the presence of VUR may result in pyelonephritis. If UTI is suspected, urinalysis and urine culture should be obtained prior to the study, and antibiotics should be initiated before proceeding. While there are no standard recommendations for how long to delay urodynamic studies after antibiotic treatment, it is reasonable to proceed after symptoms have subsided and urinalysis has normalized. For asymptomatic children, urine culture should be obtained on the day of the procedure for potential bacterial speciation and antibiotic sensitivity in the case of UTI after the study. The administration of prophylactic antibiotics after urodynamics has been found to reduce significant bacteriuria when compared to placebo (4 % with antibiotics versus 12 % without, risk ratio (RR) 0.35, 95 % CI 0.22–0.56) in adults. However, studies have found no statistically significant difference in the risk of fever, dysuria, or adverse reactions [10].

Communication with the patient's family the week prior to the study to query about symptoms of constipation and UTI, initiate therapy if indicated, and ensure withholding or taking of medications as indicated, is often invaluable to the conduct of an accurate study.

The Urodynamic Room

A child-friendly atmosphere is of upmost importance when performing urodynamics in children. Bright colors, cartoon characters, and cheerful decorations create a relaxing and familiar surrounding for children. Comfortable child-friendly gowns and socks should be provided to prevent soiling of clothing. Toys with motion, lights, or sounds are often useful to distract young children during

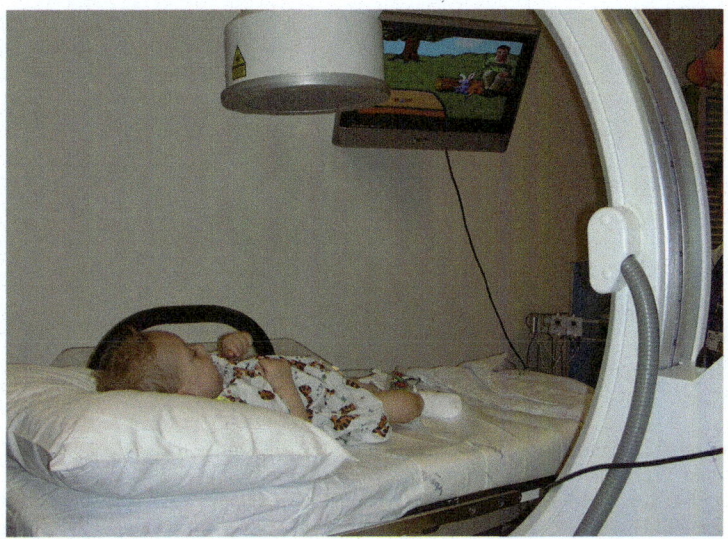

Fig. 1 Room set-up. Toddler is relaxed in supine position while watching a video. Catheters are in place. Fluoroscopy unit is in position

catheter placement and keep them entertained during the study. Music, TV/video, or gaming systems can help combat anxiety or boredom in older children (Fig. 1). The promise of a trip to a treasure box of toys after the study can encourage participation and reward a child for tolerating the invasive study. For infants, having bottles available for feeding can be calming.

An experienced team of professionals who are comfortable working with children is the cornerstone to a well-performed urodynamics study. Nursing staff that are welcoming to children, competent in pediatric catheter placement, and well-versed in the urodynamic set up will decrease stress for the family and child, as well as the time to conduct the study. More than one staff member may be required for a second pair of hands, especially in younger children who may be uncooperative and move frequently, which can dislodge catheters and disrupt readings. Child Life specialists can be beneficial and should be utilized frequently, if available. Parental involvement also can alleviate the child's anxiety, and additional lead aprons are needed for them if fluoroscopy is employed.

Pre-study room set up is important to the efficiency of the study. If a child has the ability to void, a toilet should be prepared to allow uroflowmetry. It is often helpful to place the toilet behind a curtain to allow privacy. Preparation of appropriately selected catheters with maintenance of sterility, preparation of EMG electrodes or needles, sterile cups for urine collections, syringes, lubricant, and tape will make catheter placement and urine collection simple and efficient (Fig. 2). **All equipment, including computerized urodynamic equipment and fluoroscopy unit, if utilized, should be ready with all connections made and functionality tested prior to patient arrival**. A special radiolucent table that can be moved into the sitting position is necessary if fluoroscopy is utilized.

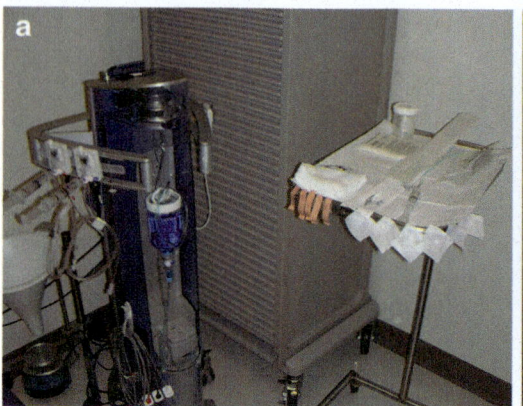 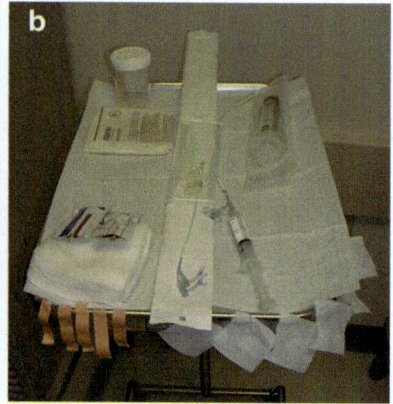

Fig. 2 Set-up for efficient patient preparation for study. (**a**) Urodynamics tower has been prepared with Pabd and Pves transducers primed with fluid. Note the *blue dye* added to bottle of radio-opaque contrast. Nearby prep table is readied with necessary supplies. (**b**) Prep tablet has both *pink plastic tape* to hold catheters to penis/legs, and cloth tape to cover EMG electrodes, antiseptic and adhesive solution swabs, gauze for drying, urethral dual lumen catheter with lubricant, rectal catheter with priming syringe, sterile gloves, sterile container for urine culture, and large syringe for bladder aspiration

For the sensate child or the child familiar with medical settings, catheter placement often creates the greatest anxiety and barrier to cooperation. Placement of a small amount of lidocaine 2 % jelly to the urethral meatus for a few minutes will provide an anesthetic effect and may reduce both the child's anxiety and the initial discomfort of the catheter placement. For older boys, instillation of the jelly into the urethra with a nozzle tip can further ease the trauma of catheter insertion. Occasionally, some children are uncooperative regardless of efforts to decrease stress, and sedation or mask anesthesia for catheter and electrode placement may be necessary with urodynamics performed once the child has recovered and is fully awake. Midazolam or low-dose ketamine have been shown to provide satisfactory sedation during pediatric urodynamic studies without impacting urodynamic values [11]. Rarely, if children are combative, urodynamics may be performed under general anesthesia. **However, urodynamics performed in a fully anesthetized child may be inaccurate and will not allow any assessment of voiding.**

Catheter and EMG Placement

Prior to catheter and EMG placement, uroflowmetry should be performed in patients who are able to volitionally void. This differentiates pediatric urodynamics from adults because many children studied are not able to void volitionally—either because of age or the high proportion with neurogenic bladder. Parents should be instructed to adequately hydrate the child and prevent voiding while waiting for the study to begin. A bladder scan can be utilized to measure the pre-void urinary volume. While the current International Children's Continence Society recommendations are for examination of PVR after uroflowmetry with ultrasonography [12], in the setting of urodynamics, the PVR may be measured when the urodynamic catheters are placed. Uroflowmetry may only be accurate when the voided volume is greater than 50 % of the maximum bladder volume [13]. The uroflow curve pattern should be noted, and specific types are well described [14].

All children are initially placed in the supine position for catheter and EMG probe placement. Infants, and toddlers remain in the supine position for the study as do some older children with neuropathies that prevent stability in the sitting position. While children should never be restrained, it is sometimes necessary to gently hold the lower extremities while parents help secure the upper body of the child. Children who are large enough and can void volitionally are then moved in the sitting position. This allows the child to void in a more natural position and into the collection funnel during the voiding component of the study. It is rare to conduct a study in the standing position in children. The child and equipment (particularly the C-arm, if fluoroscopy is used) should be positioned so that urinary leakage during detrusor contractions or movement is easily detectable. It is helpful to place a small amount of methylene blue or indigo carmine into the filling solution and a white gauze near the urethral meatus to better detect leakage.

Electromyography (EMG) monitoring of the pelvic floor and external sphincter can be done non-invasively via patch EMG surface electrodes or invasively via needle electrodes. These are typically placed at the 3 and 9 o'clock positions around the anal sphincter since its innervation and function is in parallel with the external urethral sphincter [1]. Patch surface electrodes are more easily and painlessly placed and, therefore, commonly used in children. For these, one should wipe the perineum clean, apply a skin adhesive (such as tincture of benzoin), and cover the patches with tape to prevent EMG artifact if they get wet with voiding, particularly if the child is supine (Fig. 3). Needle EMG is performed using a 24 gauge needle electrodes. Consideration of their use is a trade-off between their more invasive and threatening nature to a child versus their providing more accurate information on sphincter activity during bladder filling and emptying [15].

Urodynamic catheter size and type should be based on the child's size and the questions to be answered by the study. **In children a 6 Fr, 7 Fr, or 8 Fr dual lumen urethral catheter without a balloon is standard with smaller catheters used in smaller children, especially boys**. Since different sized catheters may be used in multiple studies over the course of the day, technical adjustments of the pump may be required. Triple lumen catheters with an occlusion balloon to obstruct the bladder neck may be needed in cases of severe urethral incompetency. This is particularly important when planning bladder outlet surgery because, without occlusion, determination of maximal bladder capacity and pressures and the need for bladder augmentation may be inaccurate.

The bladder must be emptied after the catheter is placed into the bladder. Return of urine confirms proper placement, but no urine may be present if pre-study voiding

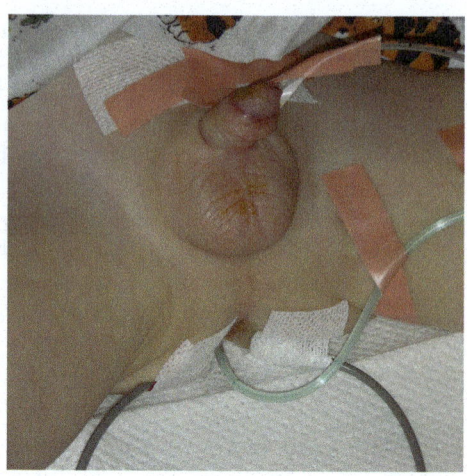

Fig. 3 Toddler male with catheters in place. *Pink plastic tape* is placed longitudinally on penis and urethral catheter after application of adhesive solution. This is further secured to lower abdominal wall. Rectal catheter is taped to inner thigh. EMG electrodes are placed peri-anally at 3 and 9 o'clock and covered with cloth tape

was complete. A bladder ultrasound (or BladderScan) may be helpful to determine if the bladder is truly empty. The residual volume is recorded. In patients that do not void, it may be faster to empty the bladder first with a larger single lumen catheter before placing the urodynamic catheter.

Rectal catheters typically measure 6–7 Fr and may be dual lumen with a balloon to detect pressure. The catheters are typically inserted 3–4 cm; however, if anal sphincter laxity is obvious (in children with low spinal lesions or history of imperforate anus surgery), inserting the catheter further may prevent expulsion of the catheter with movement or rectal contraction. In the child with an imperforate or atretic anus, the catheter may need to be placed in the colostomy to detect abdominal pressure. Having the child cough or Valsalva or pressing on the abdomen in those unable to cooperate to insure proper pressure detection in both the bladder (Pves) and rectal (Pabd) catheters is crucial before proceeding further. Special attention is required in children with neurogenic bladder who are often constipated, as mentioned previously.

Securing the catheters is perhaps one of the most critical steps in performing accurate urodynamics in children. For boys, it is most easily accomplished by placing a clear adhesive bandage around or tape along the length of the penis and catheter (Fig. 3). For girls, either can be used to secure the catheter to the upper inner thigh near the perineum to prevent dislodgement with movement. Rectal catheters should be secured similarly to the inner aspect of the gluteal crease. Regardless of the technique utilized, the catheters should double checked to ensure the child is unable to dislodge the catheter with movement or by grabbing and pulling.

If fluoroscopy is utilized, C-arm positioning must be considered so that all catheters and the meatus can be visualized and that the unit be adjusted to image both the upper and lower urinary tract during the study. In infants, this is relatively simple since they are supine and little adjustment is needed to image the entire urinary tract. However, in older children in the sitting position, greater adjustments will be required to allow proper visualization of the bladder neck, especially during voiding, while having the flexibility to image the upper tracts to rule out VUR. It cannot be emphasized enough to limit radiation exposure in children, as gonadal irradiation is unavoidable. No standard recommendations exist for the number of images, but images at the initiation of filling, at half and full capacity and during voiding should be obtained. While the average effective dose of ionizing radiation from videourodynamics is less compared to VCUG, exposure is dependent on fluoroscopy time, body mass index and bladder capacity [16].

The Study

Filling Cystometry

Expected bladder capacity should be determined prior to initiating the study. There are various equations for determining expected bladder capacity. Age + 2 (× 30 ml) is the most widely accepted formula for determining expected bladder capacity; however, for children that are significantly large or small for age, that may need to be adjusted by considering their weight on a standard somatic growth chart. Under the age of 2 years, an alternative formula is weight in kg. × 7 ml. Bladder filling with injection pumps should be performed at a rate of 5–10 % of the expected bladder capacity per minute [17]. Alternatively, fluid can be hung 30–40 cm above the level of the bladder, and a gravity drip can be used [18]. There is little agreement on whether to use solution at room temperature or heated to body temperature via a water bath in efforts to reduce bladder irritability [19]. At the onset of filling, a quick fluoroscopic image is helpful to determine proper positioning of the C-arm and bladder catheter. Faint appearance of the contrast may suggest incomplete bladder emptying during set-up. If fluoroscopy is not utilized, sonography can be used to monitor bladder filling. Periodically, the child should be asked to cough or one should push on the suprapubic area to ensure all monitors are continuing to detect pressure properly. For older children, the initiation of filling may create an unusual sensation, resulting in anxiety with the report of the need to void after minimal volume. Encouragement will usually convince the child to allow additional filling.

    Throughout the filling phase, detrusor pressures should be closely monitored. A normal bladder should fill with minimal pressure changes. Intermittent changes in detrusor pressures >15 cm H_2O above baseline are indicative of detrusor overactivity, also referred to as uninhibited bladder contractions, and these contractions may increase in both frequency and magnitude as bladder volume increases [12]. **If detrusor overactivity or rapid rise in pressure is noted, the infusion rate should be lowered. Often, decreasing the rate by 50 % or more can alleviate detrusor contractions or demonstrate more realistic compliance and provide a study more representative of natural bladder filling** (Fig. 4a, b).

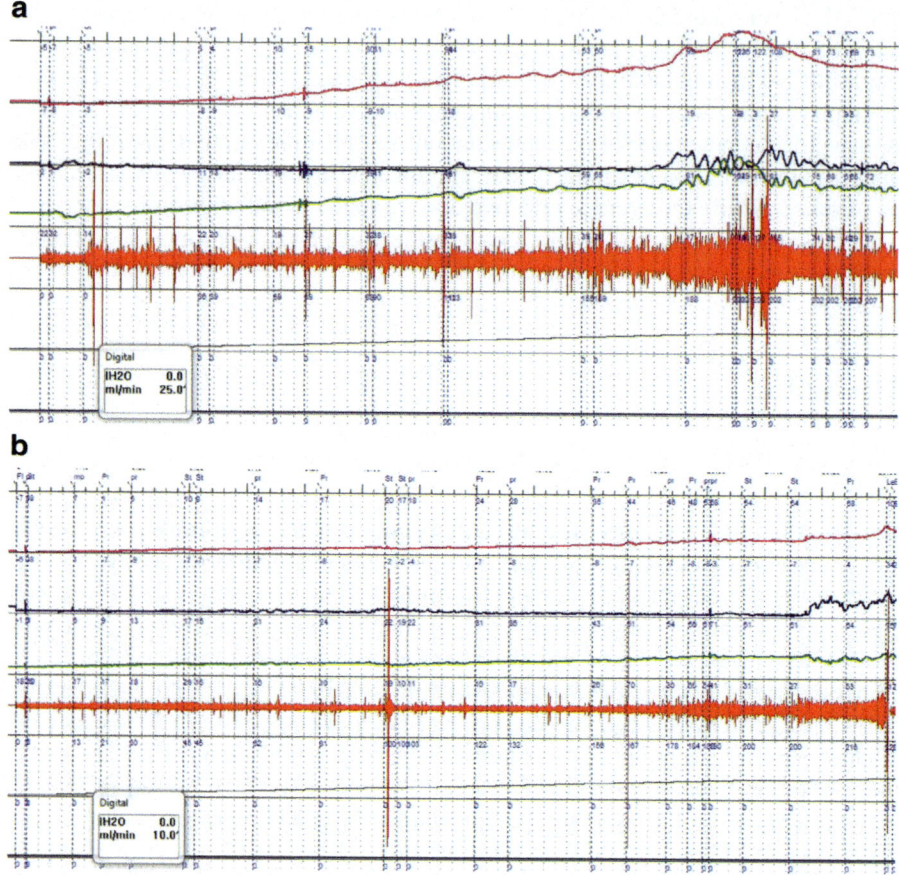

Fig. 4 Effect of filling rate on pressure curves. (**a**) Fill rate of 25 ml/min. Pves (*magenta*) shows steady rise followed by a contraction with peak pressure of 136 cm H_2O at volume of 202 ml (*black line* on fifth row). Pabd (*dark blue*) shows rectal contractions near end of filling, and these negatively affect Pdet tracing (*green*). EMG tracing (*red*) shows increased activity as detrusor contaction occurs just before volume reaches 188 ml, reflective of detrusor sphincter dyssynergia. (**b**) A second infusion at 10 ml/min is performed immediately following the previous study. Similar capacity is noted with detrusor contraction at 228 ml. Rise in pressure is diminished at this fill rate. Increased sphincter EMG activity is seen with increasing volume and detrusor pressure; dyssynergia is then noted with detrusor contraction. The increase in Pabd (*dark blue*) near capacity is not associated with patient movement and again represents rectal contraction and is subtracted from Pdet (*green*)

In older children, sensation can be monitored by recording the first and additional sensing of filling as well as the urge to void. Abdominal pressure should also be closely watched as some children with neuropathic bowel will have uninhibited rectal contractions during filling, and this will create artifact in the detrusor pressure which is the difference between bladder and rectal (abdominal) pressures.

Bladder capacity is one of the key parameters to evaluate bladder function, so the child should be encouraged to allow filling to occur as long as possible. Distraction tools mentioned previously may take the child's mind off of the bladder and allow higher volumes to be achieved. Filling should continue until the child has a strong urge to void, micturition occurs, or the child is uncomfortable [14]. For children that cannot communicate verbally, one must closely observe the child for signs of restlessness or abdominal distension. In children with poor sensation, severe VUR, or inability to void, filling should be stopped at 150–200 % of expected bladder capacity, with prolonged detrusor pressure >40 cm H_2O, or the child is uncomfortable or agitated [1]. Children with neurogenic bladder may have absent or altered sensation in which bladder fullness is manifested as abdominal fullness or back pain. In those with incontinence due to high detrusor pressure and/or incompetent outlet, filling may be stopped when the rate of leakage appears to equal the infusion rate.

Bladder compliance is another critical parameter of bladder function. Compliance can be measured as an absolute detrusor pressure at capacity or as a ratio of volume/pressure (ml/cm of H_2O). A normally compliant bladder should store a given volume of urine at a low pressure. While there are no standard reference values for safe compliance in children, investigators have reported that normal compliance is detrusor pressure ≤10 cm H_2O at capacity [12]. When compliance is decreased and detrusor pressure rises, sphincter function plays an important role in determining bladder hostility and potential for upper tract deterioration. This is evaluated by determining the pressure at which incontinence is noted (detrusor leak point pressure=DLPP) If the urethral sphincter is incompetent and DLPP is low, urine leaks out before bladder pressures become deleterious. **If the sphincter is competent and does not allow leakage of urine at all or until higher pressures are reached, the DLPP will be higher (or not existent if leakage does not occur), as will the risk to the upper tracts. A cut-off point for bladder hostility of DLPP>40 cm H_2O is based upon McGuire's classic work correlating with upper tract damage in spina bifida patients** [20].

Abdominal (previously called Valsalva or stress) leak point pressure is the pressure at which incontinence is noted when abdominal pressure is increased by coughing, straining, talking, laughing, or pushing up on the table in cooperative children or by crying, verbalizations, movement, or pressing on the suprapubic area in infants and uncooperative children. This is measure of urethral competency and is less a reflection of detrusor function.

Voiding Cystometry

The voiding phase is an integral part of urodynamic evaluation and can be augmented by fluoroscopic imaging of the bladder and bladder neck. **The voiding phase is less commonly obtained in children than in adults because a higher proportion of studies are in children that are unable or unwilling to void**

during the evaluation. Voiding pressure may vary based on age and gender of the child. Typically, voiding pressures are higher when the urethra is smaller, as noted in infants relative to older children. The same is true in boys relative to girls, by about 5–15 cm of H_2O [21, 22]. It is unclear how much the presence of a catheter may affect voiding pressures in a small urethra.

Rarely, children are unwilling or scared to void on the special table or with the fluoroscopy unit present and may benefit from moving carefully to a toilet seat with catheters in place; changes in pressures due to repositioning must be noted. If the child is unable to void around the urodynamic catheter either due to catheter obstruction of the urethra or due to a poorly contractile bladder that cannot overcome minimal urethral obstruction, voiding is sometimes achieved by removing the urethral catheter. In this case, the EMG leads or needles should be left in place to assess sphincteric function during voiding. Although voiding pressures are obviously lost, the flow rate and flow curve pattern are helpful.

There are technical challenges of collecting urine in the supine position or even in the sitting position in small children, so flow studies cannot always be obtained. In older children, flow rates vary by gender and age. In one study, children aged 5–10 years had maximum and mean flow rates of 15.26 ± 4.54 ml/s and 7.68 ± 3.26 ml/s , respectively, for boys and 17.98 ± 6.06 ml/s and 9.19 ± 4.23 ml/s, respectively, for girls. For older children, aged 11–15 years, rates were 22.50 ± 7.24 ml/s and 10.78 ± 4.03 ml/s, respectively, for boys and 27.16 ± 9.37 ml/s and 13.48 ± 5.21 ml/s, respectively, for girls [23]. The flow rates and curve pattern may be affected by neuropathic and non-neuropathic sphincteric dysfunction and by anatomic obstruction. Imaging during videourodynamics can be very helpful in these instances. Low voiding pressures with slow or poor flow curves suggest an underactive detrusor; whereas, high voiding pressures with slow or poor flow curves are indicative of anatomical or functional urethral obstruction. The normal flow curve should be bell-shaped. Abnormal patterns include tower shaped (overactive detrusor), staccato (intermittent sphincter overactivity or dysfunctional voiding), interrupted (detrusor underactivity with abdominal straining or poor detrusor/sphincter coordination) or plateau (underactive bladder or functional/anatomic urethral obstruction) [14]. Combining this information with readings of abdominal pressure and sphincter EMG activity during voiding can aid in diagnosis. Significant increases in urethral sphincter function during uninhibited bladder contractions are indicative of detrusor-sphincter dyssynergia and can result in hostile bladder pressures. It can be difficult to differentiate sphincteric activity from artifact due to crying or movement in an uncooperative child, and needle EMG electrodes may be superior in this aspect.

Finally, the residual urine should be noted by imaging, if used, and confirmed by aspiration of bladder catheter before removal. This value should be compared with the pre-study PVR to see if the presence of the catheter during voiding affected emptying.

Special Populations

Neural Tube Defects

The most common cause of neurogenic bladder are neural tube defects of which 85 % are due to myelomeningocele [24]. Patients with lipomyelomeningocele, tethered cord, occult spinal dysraphism, sacral agenesis, imperforate anus or other anorectal malformations and spinal cord injury may also have similarly significantly abnormal bladder function. The most common findings are detrusor/sphincter synergy (26 %), dyssynergy with and without poor detrusor compliance (37 %), and complete denervation (36 %) [21]. For this reason, baseline studies are recommended soon after birth or when diagnosis is made. **Clearly, not all children with neuropathic bladders will have a hostile bladder and be at risk for upper tract deterioration, but it is imperative to identify those children with significant risk factors such a poorly compliant bladder with or without sphincter dyssynergia, DLPP>40 cm H_2O, or voiding pressures over 80–100 cm H_2O** [1]. Studies have shown that early intervention in neonates with hostile bladder and sphincter activity improves long term outcome [9]. While an exact algorithm for interval urodynamic evaluation in these children does not exist, it is recommended to repeat urodynamics yearly initially during the period of rapid growth with less frequent studies as the child ages and becomes able to report changes in symptoms. Urodynamic evaluation is also recommended if changes in urologic symptoms such as recurrent UTI or new onset of urinary incontinence occur or if changes in neurological function or orthopedic examination are detected. Additionally, regular renal imaging is imperative for early detection of increased dilation of the kidney or ureter which may be indicative of deterioration in bladder function and warrant repeat urodynamics.

Posterior Urethral Valve

Posterior urethral valve is the most common cause of lower urinary obstruction in boys. Due to presence of obstruction during fetal development of the bladder, abnormal bladder function is common even after ablation of the valve. Eighty percent of infant boys will demonstrate abnormal bladder function, most commonly poor bladder compliance and detrusor overactivity with abnormal sphincter function on urodynamic evaluation [25]. The high pressures can have devastating effects on the already altered kidneys with an increasing rate of renal failure with age [26]. Over time, the bladder often changes with reduction in filling pressure and overactivity towards increasing bladder capacity and potential emptying difficulties representing eventual myogenic failure [25]. Urodynamics is an important objective measure of the function of the valve bladder and allows targeted management which may help obtain continence and protect tenuous renal function.

Bladder Exstrophy

There is a wide variation in outcomes following repair of bladder exstrophy. Continence after primary closure is possible, although bladder capacity may be decreased. Compliance is usually normal, but unstable contractions may be present in 21–67 % of patients [27, 28]. Bladder capacity may increase from a third to one-half of the predicted volume for age with approximately 80 % of patients maintaining compliant and stable bladders without bladder neck reconstruction [28]. Urodynamics is integral to the evaluation of the incontinent exstrophy patient. The urethral meatus may be difficult to locate in some cases, requiring catheter placement with sedation or placement of an SP tube. Bladder instability or mild decreases in compliance may be treated medically; whereas, inadequate bladder capacity and weak outlet noted by low LPP likely require bladder augmentation and bladder outlet procedures, respectively [28]. Even after bladder neck reconstruction that was considered successful, voiding is rarely normal with clinical and urodynamic voiding abnormalities noted in 72 % [29].

Voiding Dysfunction

Most children with voiding symptoms such as urinary urgency, frequency, or incontinence, coupled with nocturnal enuresis, recurrent UTIs, and/or constipation and fecal incontinence will respond to conservative measures including behavioral, medical, and pelvic floor therapy/biofeedback. **Urodynamics should be reserved for the minority of children with voiding dysfunction who fail conservative therapy or those with neurologic signs or symptoms**. In this select population, urodynamics will often reveal a variation of voiding abnormalities including reduced bladder capacity, detrusor overactivity, sphincteric dysfunction, infrequency voiding (lazy bladder syndrome) or psychological non-neuropathic bladder (Hinman's Syndrome) [30].

Those with small capacity bladders may have elevated detrusor filling pressures and a strong urge to void with uninhibited contractions [30]. A spinning top urethra (Fig. 5) may indicate failure of the external sphincter to relax. Detrusor overactivity is noted during the filling phase and may not be noted by the child or present as urgency and/or incontinence. The lazy bladder syndrome manifests clinically as infrequent voiding and will typically show a large bladder capacity with high PVR. In some cases, detrusor contractions are absent but in most cases, EMG activity is typically normal [30, 31].

One of the most concerning abnormality found in children is psychological non-neuropathic bladder or Hinman's Syndrome. Voiding is hindered by significant contractions of the external sphincter, resulting in functional obstruction. Children with Hinman's syndrome have urinary systems with changes similar to the neurogenic bladder. Severe hydroureteronephrosis with or without VUR, trabeculated bladders

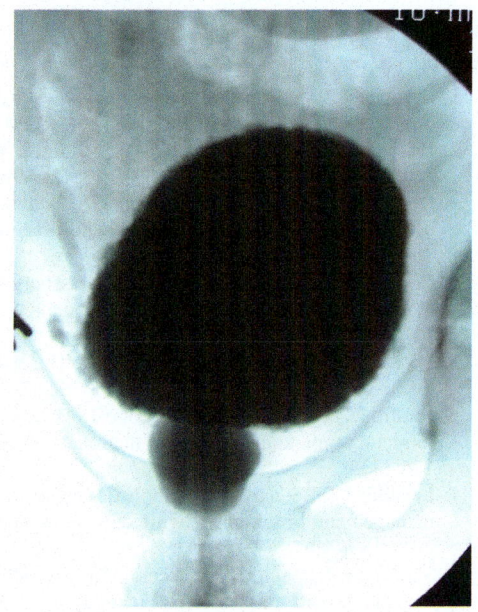

Fig. 5 Fluoroscopic image of bladder with spinning top urethra. The urethra is dilated between the bladder neck and external sphincter. Bladder trabeculation and vesicoureteral reflux into the distal right ureter are seen as well

with large capacity, and high PVR are common. Urodynamics often reveal large capacity bladders that are poorly compliant with detrusor overactivity, and high pressure voiding with reduced flow rates due to the lack of sphincter relaxation [30]. With time, myogenic failure may occur with ineffective or absent bladder contractions.

Conclusion

Urodynamics is a useful tool in the armamentarium of the pediatric urologist and its mandatory usage in the neurogenic bladder population insures detection of hostile bladders that can lead to upper tract damage. It is also helpful in attainment of continence in these patients and in those with urethral valves and bladder exstrophy. While it should be used sparingly in the non-neurogenic bladder population, it may be helpful when conservative management has failed. In all cases, a child friendly atmosphere and an experienced team who can adapt to children of different ages, sizes, and ability to cooperate is necessary. Careful observation during each phase of the study is imperative to understanding function and coordination between the bladder and sphincter. Pathological abnormalities of special populations require tailoring each study to the specific needs of each child.

References

1. Drzewiecki BA, Bauer SB. Urodynamic testing in children: indications, technique, interpretation and significance. J Urol. 2011;186(4):1190–7.
2. Hoebeke P, Bower W, Combs A, De Jong T, Yang S. Diagnostic evaluation of children with daytime incontinence. J Urol. 2010;183(2):699–703.
3. Desantis DJ, Leonard MP, Preston MA, Barrowman NJ, Guerra LA. Effectiveness of biofeedback for dysfunctional elimination syndrome in pediatrics: a systematic review. J Pediatr Urol. 2011;7(3):342–8.
4. Combs AJ, Van Batavia JP, Chan J, Glassberg KI. Dysfunctional elimination syndromes–how closely linked are constipation and encopresis with specific lower urinary tract conditions? J Urol. 2013;190(3):1015–20.
5. Combs AJ, Glassberg AD, Gerdes D, Horowitz M. Biofeedback therapy for children with dysfunctional voiding. Urology. 1998;52:312–5.
6. Kaufman MR, DeMarco RT, Pope IV JC, et al. High yield of urodynamics performed for refractory nonneurogenic dysfunctional voiding in the pediatric population. J Urol. 2006; 176:1835.
7. Lavallée LT, Leonard MP, Dubois C, Guerra LA. Urodynamic testing—is it a useful tool in the management of children with cutaneous stigmata of occult spinal dysraphism? J Urol. 2013;189(2):678–83.
8. Scottoni F, Iacobelli BD, Zaccara AM, Totonelli G, Schingo AM, Bagolan P. Spinal ultrasound in patients with anorectal malformations: is this the end of an era? Pediatr Surg Int. 2014; 30(8):829–31.
9. Edelstein RA, Bauer SB, Kelly MD, et al. The long-term urological response of neonates with myelodysplasia treated proactively with intermittent catheterization and anticholinergic therapy. J Urol. 1995;154:1500.
10. Foon R., Toozs-Hobson, Latthe P. Prophylactic antibiotic to reduce the risk of urinary tract infections after urodynamic studies. Cochran Database Syst Rev. 2012 Oct 17;10..
11. Thevaraja AK, Batra YK, Rakesh SV, Panda NB, Rao KL, Chhabra M, Aggarwal M. Comparison of low-dose ketamine to midazolam for sedation during pediatric urodynamic study. Paediatr Anaesth. 2013;23(5):415–21.
12. Nevéus T, von Gontard A, Hoebeke P, et al. The standardization of terminology of lower urinary tract function in children and adolescents: report from the Standardisation Committee of the International Children's Continence Society. J Urol. 2006;176:314.
13. Nijman RJM, Bower W, Butler U, et al. Diagnosis and management of urinary incontinence and encopresis in childhood. In: Abrams P, Cardozo L, Khoury S, et al., editors. 3rd international consultation on incontinence. Paris: Health Publications; 2005. p. 967–1057.
14. Austin PF, Bauer SB, Bower W, Chase J, Franco I, Hoebeke P, Rittig S, Vande Walle J, von Gontard A, Wright A, Yang SS, Neveus T. The standardization of terminology of lower urinary tract function in children and adolescents: update report from the standardization committee of the International Children's Continence Continence Society. J Urol. 2014;191:1863–5.
15. Bauer SB. Neurogenic bladder: etiology and assessment. Pediatr Nephrol. 2008;23:541.
16. Hsi RS, Dearn J, Dean M, Zamora DA, Kanal KM, Harper JD, Merguerian PA. Effective and organ specific radiation doses from videourodynamics in children. J Urol. 2013;190(4):1364–9.
17. Hjalmas K. Urodynamics in normal infants and children. Scand J Urol Nephrol Suppl. 1988;114:20.
18. Guerra L, Leonard M, Castagnetti M. Best practice in the assessment of bladder function in infants. Ther Adv Urol. 2014;6(4):148–64.
19. Bael A, Lax H, de Jong TP, Hoebeke P, Nijman RJ, Sixt R, Verhulst J, Hirche H, van Gool JD, European Bladder Dysfunction Study (European Union BMH1-CT94-1006). The relevance of urodynamic studies for Urge syndrome and dysfunctional voiding: a multicenter controlled trial in children. J Urol. 2008;180(4):1486–93.

20. McGuire EJ, Woodside JR, Borden TA, Weiss RM. The prognostic value of urodynamic testing in myelodysplastic patients. J Urol. 1981;126:205–9.
21. Yeung CK, Sihoe JDY, Bauer SB. Voiding dysfunction in children: non-neurogenic and neurogenic. In: Wein AJ, Kavoussi LR, Novick AC, et al., editors. Campbell-Walsh urology. 9th ed. Philadelphia, PA: Saunders Elsevier; 2007. p. 3604–55.
22. Sillén U. Bladder dysfunction and vesicoureteral reflux. Adv Urol. 2008;815472. doi:10.1155/2008/815472. Epub 2008 Nov 4.
23. Gupta DK, Sankhwar SN, Goel A. Uroflowmetry nomograms for healthy children 5 to 15 years old. J Urol. 2013;190(3):1008–13. doi:10.1016/j.juro.2013.03.073.
24. Bauer SB, Austin PF, Rawashdeh YF, de Jong TP, Franco I, Siggard C, Jorgensen TM. International Children's Continence Society's recommendation for initial diagnostic evaluation and follow-up in congenital neuropathic bladder and bowel dysfunction in children. Neurourol Urodyn. 2012;31:610–4.
25. Ghanem MA, Wolffenbuttel KP, De Vylder A, et al. Long-term bladder dysfunction and renal function in boys with posterior urethral valves based on urodynamic findings. J Urol. 2004; 171:2409.
26. Woodhouse CRJ. The fate of the abnormal bladder in adolescence. J Urol. 2001;166:2396.
27. Hollowell JG, Hill PD, Duffy PG, et al. Bladder function and dysfunction in exstrophy and epispadias. Lancet. 1991;338:926.
28. Diamond DA, Bauer SB, Dinlenc C, et al. Normal urodynamics in patients with bladder exstrophy: are they achievable? J Urol. 1999;162:841.
29. Yerkes EB, Adams MC, Rink RC, et al. How well do patients with exstrophy actually void? J Urol. 2000;164:1044.
30. Bauer S, Retik A, Colodny A, et al. The unstable bladder of childhood. Urol Clin North Am. 1980;7:321.
31. Webster G, Koefoot R, Sihelnic S. Urodynamic abnormalities in neurologically normal children with micturition dysfunction. J Urol. 1984;132:74.

Index

A

Abdominal leak point pressure (ALPP), 55
Abrams-Griffiths nomogram, 115, 120
    bladder outlet obstruction, 114, 115
    detrusor pressure, 114
    post-operative pressure-flow curve, 115
    pressure-flow plot, 114
Acetylcholine (ACh), 3
Advanced urodynamics, 10, 12, 14–17, 19
Ambulatory urodynamic monitoring (AUM)
    bladder outlet obstruction, 131
    catheters, 128, 132
    characteristics, 126–127
    definition, 126
    ICS, 127
    indications, 126
    intravesical and intra-abdominal pressures, 127
    intravesical device, 132
    leakage events, 127
    limitations, 127
    micro-tip transducer, 127–128
    natural filling, 126
    neurogenic bladder, 131, 132
    overactive bladder syndrome, 129
    remote devices, 127
    stress incontinence, 130
    valsalva maneuver, 128
    voiding occasions, 128
    vs. SU, 126
Analog signal, 18
Anticholinergic therapy, 146
Areflexic bladder, 37
AUM *See* Ambulatory urodynamic monitoring (AUM)
Autonomic nervous system, 3

B

Basic metabolic panel (BMP), 23
Basic urodynamics, 12–13, 126
BCI *See* Bladder contractility index (BCI)
Bedside urodynamics, 137, 138, 140
    catheterization, 138
    components, 136
    cystometry, 139–141
    drawback, 141
    patient selection, 136
    PVR, 138
    uroflowmetry
        average flow rate, 137
        interpretable flow test, 137
        noninvasive test, 137
        urinary stream, 138
    voiding dysfunction, 135
Benign prostatic enlargement (BPE), 67
Benign prostatic obstruction (BPO), 67, 68
Bernoulli's equation, 62, 63
Bladder contractility index (BCI), 66, 72
Bladder exstrophy, 156
Bladder neck, 94, 95, 97–99, 107, 110
Bladder outlet obstruction (BOO), 35
    AUM, 131
    females, 69–70
    fluoroscopy, 96–98
    males, 67–69
    nomograms, 114, 115, 120–123
Bladder outlet obstruction index (BOOI), 64, 65, 120, 122
Bladder overactivity (OAB), 51, 104, 114, 129
Bladder scanner, 12
Bladder ultrasonography, 138
Bladder ultrasound, 145, 150
Bladder-output relation (BOR), 65–66

BladderScan, 103, 150
Blaivas-Groutz nomogram, 120–123
BMP *See* Basic metabolic panel (BMP)

C

Carbon dioxide cystometry, 50
Catheters
  atmospheric cap, 46
  AUM, 128
  in children, 148–151
  pressure transducer, 46
  stopcock, 46
  urodynamics labs, 47
Catheter-tip transducer, 44
Concentric needle electrodes (CNE), EMG, 78
Condom catheter method (CCM), 39
Cough leak point pressure (CLPP), 55
Cystografin, 50
Cystometrogram (CMG), 15, 108–110
  air-charged catheter, 44
  bladder and rectal pressures, 43
  bladder filling
    carbon dioxide cystometry, 50
    cystografin, 50
    fluoroscopy, 49
    physiologic filling, 51
    videourodynamics, 50
  BOO, 70
  catheters
    atmospheric cap, 46
    pressure transducer, 46
    stopcock, 46
    urodynamics labs, 47
  catheter-tip transducer, 44
  definition, 43
  detrusor pressure, 43, 49
  electric signal (voltage), 45
  external pressure transducer, 44
  ICS, 44
  leak point pressure, 55–56
  Micro-Tip Catheter, 44
  obstructive conditions, 45
  provocative maneuvers, 51–53
  rectal catheter, 47–48
  storage, 53, 54
  suprapubic pressure measurements, 45
  transurethral double-lumen fluid-filled catheter, 45
  troubleshooting, 56, 57
  urodynamic testing, 44, 104
  Valsalva leak point pressure, 45
  vesical pressure, 44

Cystometry
  bedside urodynamics, 139–141
  filling, 151–153
  voiding, 153–154
Cystoscopy, 10, 24, 25

D

Detrusor instability (DI), 129, 130
Detrusor leak point pressure (DLPP), 55, 153
Detrusor overactivity (DO), 52, 129–131
Detrusor pressure, 43, 49
  Abrams-Griffiths nomogram, 114, 115
  cystometry, 151, 153
  leak point pressures, 55
  PFS, 61
  vs. flow rate curves, 116, 117
Detrusor sphincter dyssynergia (DSD), 36, 83, 85
Detrusor underactivity (DU), 71, 72
Detrusor wall thickness (DWT), 38
Digital signal, 18
Dysfunctional elimination syndrome (DES), 144

E

Electrical capacitance, 33
Electromyography (EMG), 15
  CMG, 109
  CNE, 78
  concentric needles, 78
  DSD, 83
  dysfunctional voiding, 83, 84
  electrical noise, 79
  guarding reflex, 81, 82
  history of, 77–78
  infra-sacral denervation injury, 85
  in children, 148–151
  needle electrodes, 78
  neurologic conditions, 86
  neurogenic disorders, 82
  neuromodulation device, 80
  Parkinson's disease, 85
  pelvic floor muscle function, 77
  sacral injury, 85
  SNM, 80
  sphincter bradykinesia, 85
  surface electrodes, 78, 79
  technical factors, 80
  urodynamics test, 81
  valsalva/Crede voiding, 83
Electronic medical (EMR) record, 18

F

Flow controlling zone (FCZ), 63, 68
Fluid dynamics
 liquids and gasses, 5
 Pascal's Law, 5–6
Fluroscopic urodynamics (FUDS)
 See Video urodynamics (VUDS)
Fluoroscopy, 49, 70, 83
 anatomy, 92
 benefits, 107–108
 BOO, 96–98
 business models, 107
 c-arm machines, 106
 contrast media, 98, 99
 costs and effort, 106
 facility requirements, 91
 incontinence, 95
 licensing, 90
 lower urinary tract, 90
 machine requirements, 91
 physical plant, 106
 post-void image, 94
 radiation safety, 91–92
 radiographic study, 92
 resting image, 93
 scout film, 93
 strain (Valsalva)/cough image, 94
 troubleshooting, 99
 VCUG, 94, 96
Food and Drug Administration (FDA), 91

H

Hyperglycemia, 102

I

International Consultation of Incontinence Questionnaire Short Form on Urinary Incontinence (ICIQ-UI), 22
International Continence Society (ICS), 44, 126
 AUM, 127, 128
 guidelines, 47
 nomogram, 118–120, 122
 recommendation, 45
 terminology, 63
Interstitial cystitis/bladder pain syndrome (IC/BPS), 51, 53
Intravesical pressure, 48, 57, 99, 111
Israeli urogynecologist Asnat Groutz, 121

L

LaPlace's Law, 7
Leak point pressure, 55–56, 95, 110, 153
Linearized passive urethral relation curve (LinPURR), 117
Lower urinary tract
 anatomy, 1, 2
 biomechanics, 6–7
 fluoroscopy, 90
 function, 1, 31
 neural control
  ACh, 3
  autonomic nervous system, 3
  bladder filling, 3
  longitudinal muscle layers, 4
  micturition event, 4
  postganglionic parasympathetic neurons, 3
  purposes of, 3
  urethra-spinal-bladder reflex, 4
  urethra-spinal-urethra reflex, 4
  urethra-spinobulbospinal-bladder reflex, 4
Lower urinary tract symptoms (LUTS), 26, 97, 114
PFS, 67
UFM, 32

M

Microscopic hematuria, 23
Micro-Tip Catheter, 44
Micro-tip transducer, 127, 128
Motor unit potential (MUP), 85
Multi-channel urodynamics, 92

N

Near infrared spectroscopy (NIRS), 39
Neural control
 ACh, 3
 autonomic nervous system, 3
 bladder filling, 3
 longitudinal muscle layers, 4
 micturition event, 4
 postganglionic parasympathetic neurons, 3
 purposes of, 3
 urethra-spinal-bladder reflex, 4
 urethra-spinal-urethra reflex, 4
 urethra-spinobulbospinal-bladder reflex, 4
Neural tube defects, 155
Neurogenic bladder, 26, 110, 131, 132, 144–145

Neurologic disease, 21
NIU *See* Noninvasive urodynamics (NIU)
Nomograms
  abdominal and intravesical pressures, 67
  Abrams-Griffiths nomogram
    bladder outlet obstruction, 114, 115
    detrusor pressure, 114
    post-operative pressure-flow curve, 115
    pressure-flow plot, 114
  BCI, 66
  Bernoulli's equation, 62, 63
  bladder outlet obstruction, 120–123
  Blaivas-Groutz, 120–123
  BOOI, 64, 65
  detrusor pressure, 65, 66
  FCZ, 63
  ICS, 118–120, 122
  mathematical analysis, 62
  pressure-flow, 113
  PURR, 64
  rigid system, 63
  Schäfer nomogram, 116–119
  URR, 64
  volitional voiding, 66
Noninvasive urodynamics (NIU)
  CCM, 39
  DWT, 38
  NIRS, 39
  penile cuff test, 38
  urinary flow and bladder conditions, 31
  uroflowmetry, 31
    average flow rate, 34
    bladder function and dysfunction, 32
    BOO, 35
    continuous flow curves, 35
    dysfunctional voiding, 35
    electrical capacitance, 33
    flow rate, 34
    flow time, 34
    indications, 32
    intermittent flow curve, 36
    maximum flow rate, 34
    normal curve, 35
    preparation, 33
    PVR, 34, 37
    rotating disc, 33
    technique, 34
    time to maximum flow, 34
    toy erector set, 32
    urine flow rate, 32, 34
    voided volume, 34
    voiding time, 34
    weight, 33
Non-neurogenic bladder, 143, 144

O
Overactive bladder (OAB), 51, 104, 114, 129

P
Pad weight testing, 24
Parkinson's disease, 85
Pascal's Law, 5–6
Passive urethral resistance relation (PURR), 64, 116, 118
Pelvic floor muscle function, 77
Penile cuff test, 38
Periprocedural antibiotic treatment, 27–28
Post void residual (PVR), 25, 34, 37, 138, 149
Posterior urethral valve, 155
Postganglionic parasympathetic neurons, 3
Pressure flow study (PFS)
  BOO
    females, 69–70
    males, 67–69
  detrusor pressure, 61
  nomograms
    abdominal and intravesical pressures, 67
    BCI, 66
    Bernoulli's equation, 62, 63
    BOOI, 64, 65
    detrusor pressure, 65, 66
    FCZ, 63
    mathematical analysis, 62
    PURR, 64
    rigid system, 63
    URR, 64
    volitional voiding, 66
  underactive detrusor contraction and valsalva voiding, 71–73
Pressure-flow nomogram, 113
Provocative maneuvers, 43, 51–53
PURR *See* Passive urethral resistance relation (PURR)
PVR *See* Post void residual (PVR)

R
Radiology, 10, 90
Rectal catheter, 47–48, 150

S
Sacral neuromodulation (SNM), 80
Schäfer nomogram, 116–119
Silver-chloride surface electrode, 79
Sonography, 151
Speculum, 22

Index

Sphincter bradykinesia, 85
Standard urodynamic (SU) testing, 125–127
Stress urinary incontinence (SUI), 51, 53, 130
Suprapubic pressure measurements, 45

T
Triple lumen catheters, 149

U
UDS *See* Urodynamics (UDS)
UFM *See* Uroflowmetry (UFM)
Underactive detrusor contraction, 71–73
Urethral opening pressure, 62, 116
Urethral resistance relation (URR), 64
Urethral sphincter function, 146
Urethra-spinal-bladder reflex, 4
Urethra-spinal-urethra reflex, 4
Urethra-spinobulbospinal-bladder reflex, 4
Urinalysis (UA), 22
Urinary tract infections (UTI), 144–146
Urodynamics (UDS)
    advanced, 12, 14–16
    basic, 12–13
    biomechanics, 6–7
    bladder pressure curve, 108, 109
    BMP, 23
    clinical tests, 101
    CMG, 104, 108–110
    compliance, 6, 7
    correlation and clinical data, 11
    cystoscopy, 10, 24, 25
    data processing, 18
    data storage, 18
    definition, 21
    development of, 9–12
    diagnostic tests, 102
    education, 26–27
    fluid dynamics
        liquids and gasses, 5
        Pascal's Law, 5–6
    fluoroscopy
        benefits, 107–108
        business models, 107
        c-arm machines, 106
        costs and effort, 106
        physical plant, 106
    goals of, 89
    history, 21–22
    hyperglycemia, 102
    imaging studies, 25
    in children, 151
        anesthetic effect, 148
        anticholinergic therapy, 146
        bladder exstrophy, 156
        bladder function, 146
        catheter, 148–151
        child-friendly atmosphere, 146
        cystometry *see* Cystometry
        fluoroscopy, 150
        neural tube defects, 155
        neurogenic bladder, 144–145
        non-neurogenic bladder, 143, 144
        Pabd and Pves transducers, 148
        physical examination, 145
        pink plastic tape, 150
        posterior urethral valve, 155
        pre-study room set up, 147
        PVR, 149
        surface electrodes, 149
        urethral sphincter function, 146
        UTI, 146
        VCUG, 145
        voiding and stooling diary, 145
        voiding dysfunction, 156–157
    laboratory, 47, 105–106
    LaPlace's Law, 7
    lower urinary tract symptoms, 26
    neurogenic bladder dysfunction, 25
    neurogenic bladder patients, 110
    neurologic disease, 21
    non-neurogenic incontinent patients, 111
    OAB, 104
    pad weight testing, 24
    patient preparation, 26–27
    periprocedural antibiotic treatment, 27–28
    physical examination, 22
    preoperative studies, 26
    pressure flow test, 104
    PVR, 25
    radiology, 10
    room and personnel, 10, 11
    stress and strain, 7
    stress incontinence test, 104
    testing, 10, 81
    UA, 22
    uroflow and post-void residual, 103
    voiding diary, 23
    VUDS *see* Video urodynamics (VUDS)
Uroflowmetry (UFM), 12, 13, 31
    average flow rate, 34, 137
    bladder function and dysfunction, 32
    BOO, 35
    continuous flow curves, 35
    dysfunctional voiding, 35
    electrical capacitance, 33
    flow rate, 34
    flow time, 34
    indications, 32

Uroflowmetry (UFM) (*cont.*)
   intermittent flow curve, 36
   interpretable flow test, 137
   maximum flow rate, 34
   noninvasive test, 137
   normal curve, 35
   preparation, 33
   PVR, 34, 37
   rotating disc, 33
   technique, 34
   time to maximum flow, 34
   toy erector set, 32
   urinary stream, 138
   urine flow rate, 32, 34
   voided volume, 34
   voiding time, 34
   weight, 33
Urogenital Distress Inventory Short Form (UDI-6), 22
UTI *See* Urinary tract infections (UTI)

V

Valsalva leak point pressure (VLPP), 45, 55, 95, 103, 111, 153

Valsalva maneuver, 73, 81, 128
Valsalva voiding, 71–73
VCUG *See* Voiding cystourethrogram (VCUG)
Vesicoureteral reflux (VUR), 94, 107, 145, 157
Video urodynamics (VUDS), 50, 89
   BOO, 70
   components of, 12
   cystogram, 17
   fluoroscopy, 16
   lead-lined room, 17
   VCUG, 17
   vs. UDS, 17
VLPP *See* Valsalva leak point pressure (VLPP)
Voiding cystourethrogram (VCUG), 17, 94, 96, 97, 144, 145
Voiding dysfunction, 156–157
VUDS *See* Video urodynamics (VUDS)
VUR *See* Vesicoureteral reflux (VUR)

W

Watt factor (WF), 72

The manufacturer's authorised representative in the EU is Springer Nature Customer Service Centre GmbH, Europaplatz 3, 69115 Heidelberg, Germany. If you have any concerns regarding our products, please contact ProductSafety@springernature.com

Printed and bound by CPI Group (UK) Ltd, Croydon, CR0 4YY

15/08/2025

01937658-0009